# THE LOW-FODMAP DIET COOKBOOK

*The Ultimate Easy and Delicious Recipes to Soothe your Gut Health and Relieve the Symptoms of IBS*

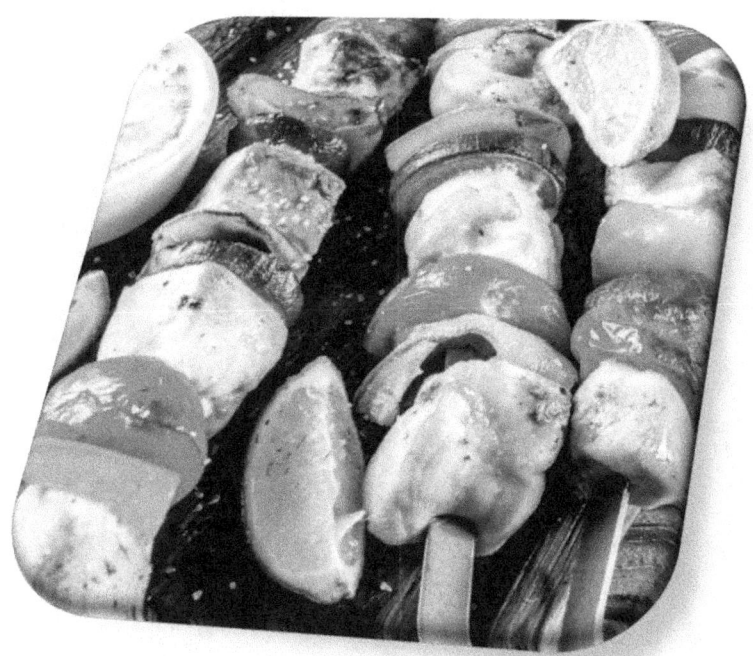

## DR. SANDRA T. CADWELL

THE LOW-FODMAP DIET COOKBOOK

# Copyright © 2024 Dr. Sandra T. Cadwell
## *All rights reserved.*

No part of this publication may be reproduced, distributed, or transmitted in any form or by any means, including photocopying, recording, or other electronic or mechanical methods, without the prior written permission of the publisher, except in the case of brief quotations embodied in critical reviews and certain other noncommercial uses permitted by copyright law.

This cookbook is a work of non-fiction. The recipes, tips, and advice provided are based on the author's experiences and research.

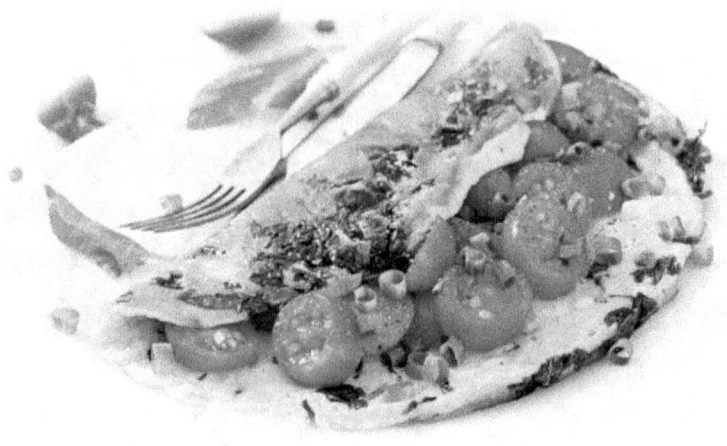

# TABLE OF CONTENTS

INTRODUCTION ................................................................. 6

    Understanding Irritable Bowel Syndrome (IBS) and Small Intestinal Bacterial Overgrowth (SIBO) ................................. 6

    Symptoms, Prevalence, and Impact on Daily Life ................. 7

    Differentiating Between IBS and SIBO .................................. 9

    What is FODMAPs? ............................................................. 10

    Role of FODMAPs in Triggering Symptoms ....................... 11

    Scientific Research-Based Evidence on Low-FODMAP Diet ............................................................................................ 12

    Guidance on Consulting with Healthcare Professionals ....... 14

    Step-by-Step Instructions for Transitioning to a Low-FODMAP Diet ..................................................................... 15

    Tips for Overcoming Common Challenges ......................... 17

CHAPTER ONE ................................................................. 20

    Understanding Your Triggers ............................................... 20

        Keeping a Food Diary and Tracking Symptoms ................... 21

        Reintroducing High-FODMAP Foods During the Challenge Phase ................................................................................... 22

    Tracking Symptoms ............................................................. 24

        Symptom Tracking Methods ................................................ 25

        Incorporating Symptom Tracking into Your Routine ........... 26

    Understanding Food Labels ................................................. 28

        How to Read Food Labels ................................................... 30

Common Hidden Sources of FODMAPs in Packaged Foods ............ 31

## CHAPTER TWO ............ 34

### Breakfast Recipes ............ 34

- Scrambled Tofu Breakfast Bowl ............ 34
- Banana Berry Smoothie Bowl ............ 36
- Quinoa Breakfast Bowl ............ 38
- Veggie Omelette ............ 40
- Peanut Butter Banana Overnight Oats ............ 42
- Spinach and Tomato Frittata ............ 44
- Lactose-Free Pancakes ............ 47
- Smoked Salmon and Dill Omelette ............ 50
- Greek Yogurt Parfait ............ 52
- Spinach and Tomato Breakfast Burrito ............ 54

## CHAPTER THREE ............ 58

### Lunch Recipes ............ 58

- Quinoa Salad with Lemon Herb Dressing ............ 58
- Grilled Chicken and Vegetable Skewers ............ 61
- Turkey and Avocado Wrap ............ 64
- Quinoa and Vegetable Stir-Fry ............ 66
- Tuna Salad Lettuce Wraps ............ 69
- Mediterranean Quinoa Salad ............ 71
- Grilled Chicken Salad with Lemon Vinaigrette ............ 73
- Eggplant and Tomato Quinoa Bowl ............ 76
- Shrimp and Vegetable Stir-Fry ............ 78

Turkey and Spinach Salad with Balsamic Vinaigrette .......... 80

CHAPTER FOUR ................................................................... 82

  Dinner Recipes ................................................................... 82

    Lemon Herb Baked Salmon ............................................. 82

    Quinoa Stuffed Bell Peppers ............................................ 84

    Chicken and Vegetable Stir-Fry ...................................... 87

    Baked Turkey Meatballs .................................................. 89

    Lemon Herb Grilled Chicken ........................................... 91

    Spaghetti Squash with Shrimp Scampi ........................... 93

    Teriyaki Glazed Salmon .................................................. 96

    Mediterranean Chicken Skewers .................................... 98

    Grilled Steak with Chimichurri Sauce ........................... 100

    Lemon Garlic Shrimp Pasta .......................................... 103

CHAPTER FIVE ................................................................... 106

  Snack Recipes ................................................................. 106

    Rice Cake with Almond Butter and Sliced Banana ........... 106

    Mixed Berry Parfait ....................................................... 108

    Veggie Sticks with Hummus .......................................... 110

    Rice Crackers with Tuna Salad ..................................... 112

    Berry Smoothie Bowl .................................................... 114

    Turkey and Cheese Roll-Ups ........................................ 116

    Cucumber and Tomato Salad ....................................... 118

    Rice Cake with Avocado and Radish ............................ 120

    Turkey and Cucumber Roll-Ups .................................... 122

    Mixed Nuts and Seeds Snack Mix ................................ 124

## CHAPTER SIX ............................................................................ 126

### Dessert Recipes .................................................................. 126

- Chocolate Banana Nice Cream ........................................... 126
- Coconut Berry Chia Pudding ............................................... 128
- Peanut Butter Banana Bites ................................................ 130
- Lemon Blueberry Yogurt Popsicles .................................... 132
- Raspberry Coconut Chia Pudding Cups ........................... 134
- Chocolate Peanut Butter Energy Balls .............................. 136
- Almond Butter Chocolate Chip Cookies ........................... 138
- Mixed Berry Frozen Yogurt Bark ........................................ 141
- Lemon Coconut Energy Bites ............................................. 143
- Chocolate Almond Butter Rice Crispy Treats .................. 145

## CHAPTER SEVEN ................................................................... 148

Shopping List ......................................................................... 148

## CONCLUSION ......................................................................... 152

# INTRODUCTION

## Understanding Irritable Bowel Syndrome (IBS) and Small Intestinal Bacterial Overgrowth (SIBO)

In terms of gastrointestinal health, two illnesses stand out as major concerns for millions of people worldwide: Irritable Bowel Syndrome (IBS) and Small Intestinal Bacterial Overgrowth (SIBO)

These medical conditions, along with their many and often baffling symptoms, throw a pall over the lives of individuals affected, disrupting their routines, social interactions, and general feeling of well-being.

Here, we will explore the complexity of IBS and SIBO, including their symptoms, prevalence, and the devastating impact they have on people's everyday lives.

IBS, also known as a functional gastrointestinal condition, is characterized by a wide range of symptoms, including abdominal discomfort, bloating, gas, diarrhea, constipation, or a combination of these.

These symptoms, which vary in strength and duration, frequently appear unexpectedly, bringing discomfort and worry to people afflicted. While the specific etiology of IBS is unknown, variables such as altered gut motility, visceral hypersensitivity, intestinal inflammation, and gut microbial dysbiosis are thought to play a role in its development.

IBS is quite common, affecting an estimated 10-15% of the global population. It has no regard for age, gender, or race, yet it typically appears in early adulthood and is more common in women.

IBS has a far-reaching impact on people's emotional and social lives. Individuals with IBS may experience worry, depression, and a worse quality of life as they deal with the problems of their illness.

SIBO, on the other hand, is a unique but interrelated concern in the field of digestive health. This disorder is defined by an overgrowth of bacteria in the small intestine, which disrupts normal digestive processes and causes a series of symptoms including bloating, stomach discomfort, diarrhea, and nutritional malabsorption.

While the precise frequency of SIBO is unknown due to diagnostic problems and differing definitions of the syndrome, it is becoming recognized as a contributor to gastrointestinal symptoms in people with underlying gut disorders.

The symptoms of SIBO sometimes coincide with those of IBS, complicating diagnosis and therapy. Individuals with SIBO may have persistent discomfort and dysfunction, limiting their ability to do everyday tasks, work, and socialize. SIBO's impact extends beyond physical symptoms, affecting nutritional status, systemic health, and overall quality of life.

## Symptoms, Prevalence, and Impact on Daily Life

IBS is a chronic functional gastrointestinal condition distinguished by a set of symptoms that include stomach pain or discomfort, bloating, gas, and changed bowel habits such as diarrhea, constipation, or a mix of the two.

These symptoms can vary in severity and length, frequently varying over time, causing substantial discomfort and a reduction in quality of life for people afflicted.

According to prevalence surveys, IBS affects between 10-15% of the global population, making it one of the most prevalent gastrointestinal illnesses. It can develop at any age, although it usually appears in early adulthood, with women being more afflicted than males.

The actual cause of IBS is unknown, however variables such as altered gut motility, visceral hypersensitivity, intestinal inflammation, and gut microbial dysbiosis are thought to play a role in its development.

Living with IBS may be difficult since symptoms are unexpected and disruptive, affecting with everyday activities, employment, social interactions, and general quality of life. Individuals with IBS may feel anxiety, sadness, and other forms of psychological distress as a result of their persistent symptoms and the ambiguity around symptom treatment.

Similarly, SIBO is a disorder characterized by bacterial overgrowth in the small intestine, which causes symptoms such as bloating, stomach discomfort, diarrhea, and nutritional malabsorption.

Excessive bacterial growth in the small intestine can disrupt normal digestion processes, causing vitamin shortages, malnutrition, and a variety of gastrointestinal symptoms.

While the exact prevalence of SIBO is difficult to determine due to diagnostic challenges and varying definitions of the condition, it is becoming more widely recognized as a contributing factor to gastrointestinal symptoms in people with IBS, inflammatory bowel disease (IBD), celiac disease, and functional dyspepsia.

SIBO can arise as a main or secondary consequence of underlying gastrointestinal diseases, resulting in overlapping symptoms and diagnostic problems.

SIBO's influence on everyday life can be significant, with symptoms ranging from mild discomfort to severe gastrointestinal distress. Individuals with SIBO may feel bloating, gas, stomach discomfort, diarrhea, and nutrient malabsorption, which can result in tiredness, weight loss, and nutritional deficits.

The chronic nature of SIBO symptoms can have a substantial impact on quality of life, including employment, social contacts, and emotional well-being.

## Differentiating Between IBS and SIBO

While IBS and SIBO have similar gastrointestinal symptoms, they are separate clinical entities with their own underlying processes and diagnostic criteria. Differentiating between the two disorders is critical for proper diagnosis and treatment.

IBS is often diagnosed based on the presence of distinctive symptoms such as stomach pain or discomfort linked with changed bowel habits, in the absence of observable structural or biochemical abnormalities.

Diagnostic criteria, such as the Rome criteria, are often used to define IBS subtypes based on predominant bowel behaviors (for example, IBS with constipation, IBS with diarrhea, or mixed IBS).

SIBO, on the other hand, is diagnosed by detecting an increased bacterial load in the small intestine, which is usually done by breath testing or aspiration culture.

Specific symptoms such as bloating, gas, and diarrhea may indicate SIBO, especially in those who have underlying gastrointestinal disorders or risk factors for bacterial overgrowth.

Despite their separate diagnostic criteria, IBS and SIBO have significant overlap, with data showing that SIBO may contribute to symptoms in a portion of IBS patients.

Individuals with IBS may be predisposed to developing SIBO due to factors such as decreased gastrointestinal motility, reduced mucosal barrier function, and gut microbial dysbiosis, which can exacerbate symptoms and contribute to diagnostic ambiguity.

Understanding the complicated interaction between IBS and SIBO is critical for healthcare practitioners to correctly diagnose and manage both illnesses.

Individuals living with IBS and SIBO require targeted diagnostic tests and personalized treatment options in order to optimize results and improve quality of life.

## What is FODMAPs?

FODMAPs, an abbreviation developed by Monash University researchers, refer to a class of short-chain carbohydrates and sugar alcohols that are poorly absorbed in the small intestine but easily digested by gut bacteria in the colon.

The acronym "FODMAP" refers to Fermentable Oligosaccharides, Disaccharides, Monosaccharides, and Polyols, each of which is a kind of carbohydrate having distinct characteristics and effects on the gastrointestinal system.

Oligosaccharides include fructans and galacto-oligosaccharides (GOS), which are present in wheat, onions, garlic, legumes, and several fruits and vegetables.

Lactose, a naturally occurring sugar found in dairy products such milk, yogurt, and soft cheeses, is an example of a disaccharide.

Monosaccharides represent fructose, a simple sugar found in fruits, honey, and high-fructose corn syrup.

Finally, polyols are sugar alcohols such as sorbitol, mannitol, xylitol, and maltitol, which are widely utilized as sweeteners in sugar-free goods and occur naturally in various fruits and vegetables.

While FODMAPs are found in a broad variety of foods, their quantity and composition vary greatly, making it difficult to pinpoint particular dietary triggers for people with IBS and SIBO.

According to research, FODMAPs have osmotic effects in the intestinal lumen, causing water to enter the colon and increase stool volume and frequency.

Furthermore, colonic bacteria metabolize undigested FODMAPs, resulting in short-chain fatty acids and gases including hydrogen, methane, and carbon dioxide, which can cause symptoms like bloating, gas, stomach discomfort, and abnormal bowel patterns.

## Role of FODMAPs in Triggering Symptoms

Consuming high-FODMAP foods can aggravate gastrointestinal symptoms and lead to illness flare-ups in people with IBS and SIBO.

The processes behind FODMAP-induced symptoms are complex, involving osmotic effects, gas generation, gut motility changes, and sensory perception changes.

Poorly absorbed FODMAPs move mainly intact through the small intestine and into the colon, where they serve as substrates for bacterial fermentation.

This fermentation process produces gasses and short-chain fatty acids, which can dilate the colon and cause symptoms including bloating, gas, and stomach pain.

Furthermore, the osmotic effects of undigested FODMAPs can cause water retention in the colon, resulting in diarrhea or loose stools in sensitive individuals.

In addition to their impact on gut physiology, FODMAPs may influence gut motility and sensory function, aggravating symptoms in people with IBS and SIBO.

Certain FODMAPs, including fructans and GOS, have been demonstrated in studies to activate colonic contractions and enhance visceral sensitivity, resulting in an increased sense of pain and discomfort in response to typical physiological stimuli.

Understanding the function of FODMAPs in triggering symptoms is critical for people with IBS and SIBO because it serves as the foundation for dietary therapies targeted at symptom management and quality of life.

Individuals who identify and restrict high-FODMAP items in their diet can lower the fermentable substrate available to colonic bacteria, alleviating FODMAP fermentation symptoms and improving overall gastrointestinal health.

## Scientific Research-Based Evidence on Low-FODMAP Diet

Numerous clinical trials and observational research have shown that the low-FODMAP diet reduces gastrointestinal symptoms and improves overall well-being in people with IBS and SIBO.

These studies have produced persuasive data supporting the significance of dietary change in symptom management, paving the path for widespread use of the low-FODMAP diet as a first-line treatment for IBS and SIBO.

Seminal research published in the Journal of Gastroenterology and Hepatology in 2017 compared the effectiveness of a low-FODMAP diet to a typical IBS diet in IBS patients.

The study discovered that people on the low-FODMAP diet had higher decreases in overall gastrointestinal symptoms, such as bloating, abdominal discomfort, and flatulence, than those on the typical IBS diet.

Those on the low-FODMAP diet reported improved quality of life and psychological well-being, emphasizing the overall advantages of dietary adjustment in controlling IBS symptoms.

Research on the impact of the low-FODMAP diet in SIBO patients has produced positive results.

A comprehensive study and meta-analysis published in the journal Clinical Gastroenterology and Hepatology in 2018 assessed the efficacy of the low-FODMAP diet in lowering SIBO symptoms and improving breath test results.

The research discovered that following a low-FODMAP diet was related with significant decreases in symptoms such as bloating, stomach discomfort, and diarrhea, as well as improvements in breath test findings indicating less bacterial overgrowth in the small intestine.

Studies have indicated that the low-FODMAP diet has benefits beyond symptom control, such as increases in overall health and well-being.

According to a study published in the journal Nutrition in Clinical Practice, following a low-FODMAP diet can reduce markers of systemic inflammation, oxidative stress, and gastrointestinal permeability, implying that dietary modification may play a role in mitigating the underlying pathophysiology of IBS and SIBO.

The evidence for the advantages of a low-FODMAP diet in controlling IBS and SIBO symptoms is strong, and it continues to develop as researchers examine the processes underlying dietary alteration and its impact on gut health. While further study is needed to understand the low-FODMAP diet's long-term benefits and durability over time, the current body of data provides convincing support for its usefulness as a therapeutic intervention for those with IBS and SIBO.

## Guidance on Consulting with Healthcare Professionals

Before making any dietary changes, contact with a healthcare expert who specializes in gastrointestinal health. A trained healthcare expert, such as a gastroenterologist, certified dietitian, or nutritionist, can guide you through the complexity of IBS and SIBO, provide specific suggestions, and track your progress along your journey.

During your session, be prepared to discuss your symptoms, medical history, dietary habits, and prior symptom management approaches. Your doctor may suggest diagnostic tests, like as breath testing for SIBO or allergy testing for food intolerances, to help discover underlying causes and guide treatment recommendations.

Furthermore, your healthcare professional may provide essential information about the low-FODMAP diet, including its possible advantages, restrictions, and long-term consequences.

They can help you set realistic objectives, answer any issues or questions you may have, and offer continuing support and encouragement as you embark on your nutritional journey.

## Step-by-Step Instructions for Transitioning to a Low-FODMAP Diet

Transitioning to a low-FODMAP diet requires careful planning, preparation, and attention to detail. Follow these step-by-step instructions to make the transition as smooth and successful as possible:

### Educate Yourself

Take the time to educate yourself about the low-FODMAP diet, its principles, and its potential impact on your symptoms. Familiarize yourself with high-FODMAP and low-FODMAP foods, as well as common sources of hidden FODMAPs in packaged and processed foods.

### Consult with a Registered Dietitian

Seek guidance from a registered dietitian who specializes in gastrointestinal health and the low-FODMAP diet. A dietitian can help you create a personalized meal plan, identify suitable alternatives for high-FODMAP foods, and address any concerns or questions you may have.

### Pantry Stocking

Clean out your pantry and refrigerator to remove high-FODMAP foods and ingredients. Stock up on low-FODMAP staples such as rice, quinoa, oats, lean proteins, low-FODMAP fruits and vegetables, lactose-free dairy products, and suitable condiments and seasonings.

### Label Reading

Develop the habit of reading food labels carefully to identify potential sources of FODMAPs in packaged and processed foods. Look for ingredients such as wheat, onions, garlic, honey, high-fructose corn syrup, and sugar alcohols, which may indicate the presence of FODMAPs.

### Meal Planning

Plan your meals and snacks in advance to ensure that they are low in FODMAPs and nutritionally balanced. Experiment with new recipes and cooking techniques to keep your meals interesting and enjoyable.

### Gradual Introduction

Gradually introduce low-FODMAP foods into your diet while reducing or eliminating high-FODMAP foods. Pay attention to how your body responds to different foods and adjust your diet accordingly based on your symptoms and tolerance levels.

### Monitor Symptoms

Keep a food diary to track your dietary intake and symptoms over time. Note any changes in symptoms, including improvements or exacerbations, and identify potential trigger foods or patterns that may be contributing to your symptoms.

## Seek Support

Lean on friends, family members, and online communities for support and encouragement as you navigate the challenges of the low-FODMAP diet. Share your experiences, recipes, and tips with others who are on a similar journey, and celebrate your successes together.

# Tips for Overcoming Common Challenges

Transitioning to a low-FODMAP diet may present various challenges, but with perseverance, patience, and creativity, you can overcome them and thrive on your dietary journey.

Here are some powerful tips for overcoming common challenges associated with the low-FODMAP diet:

## Dining Out

When dining out, research restaurant menus in advance to identify low-FODMAP options. Communicate your dietary needs to restaurant staff and ask for modifications or substitutions as needed. Focus on simple dishes made with fresh, whole ingredients, and be mindful of hidden sources of FODMAPs in sauces, dressings, and condiments.

## Social Gatherings

Navigate social gatherings with confidence by bringing your own low-FODMAP dish to share with others. Communicate your dietary needs to hosts and friends in advance, and offer to contribute to the meal planning to ensure that there are suitable options available for you to enjoy.

Focus on the company and conversation rather than the food, and prioritize your health and well-being above all else.

### *Traveling*

Prepare for travel by packing snacks and meals that are low in FODMAPs and suitable for your dietary needs. Research dining options at your destination and plan ahead to ensure that you have access to safe and nutritious food choices. Pack portable snacks such as nuts, seeds, rice cakes, and low-FODMAP fruit to keep you fueled and satisfied while on the go.

### *Stress Management*

Manage stress effectively through relaxation techniques such as deep breathing, meditation, yoga, or tai chi. Practice self-care activities that promote relaxation and well-being, such as spending time in nature, engaging in creative hobbies, or connecting with loved ones. Prioritize sleep, exercise, and stress management as integral components of your overall health and wellness routine.

### *Self-Compassion*

Be kind and sympathetic to yourself as you face the challenges of the low-FODMAP diet. Recognize that making dietary changes requires time and patience, and that setbacks are a normal part of the process.

Instead of striving for perfection, focus on making progress and celebrating minor triumphs. Treat yourself with the same compassion and understanding that you would show a friend or loved one, and remember that you are deserving of love, acceptance, and self-care.

Understanding, support, and empowerment are essential first steps in controlling irritable bowel syndrome (IBS) and small intestine bacterial overgrowth (SIBO) with dietary adjustment.

You may begin on a transforming path to digestive wellness by consulting with healthcare specialists, carefully planning and preparing for the shift to a low-FODMAP diet, and overcoming common hurdles with fortitude and inventiveness.

Prepare to take charge of your digestive health and recover your vitality, one wholesome meal at a time.

# CHAPTER ONE
## Understanding Your Triggers

This chapter delves into the notion of trigger foods, looking at typical high-FODMAP culprits, providing tips for recording symptoms, and suggesting techniques for reintroducing high-FODMAP meals during the challenge period.

By equipping yourself with information and awareness, you can discover your specific triggers, paving the path for symptom alleviation and overall well-being.

Understanding trigger foods is critical for those following the low-FODMAP diet since it serves as the foundation for dietary changes and symptom management.

Trigger foods include a high concentration of fermentable carbohydrates known as FODMAPs—short-chain carbohydrates that are poorly absorbed in the small intestine but easily fermented by gut flora in the colon.

In people with sensitive digestive systems, fermentable carbohydrates can cause symptoms such as bloating, gas, stomach discomfort, and changed bowel patterns.

### *Common high-FODMAP foods include:*

#### Fructans
Found in wheat, onions, garlic, broccoli, cauliflower, asparagus, and certain fruits such as apples and watermelon.

#### Galacto-oligosaccharides (GOS)
Present in legumes such as beans, lentils, and chickpeas, as well as certain nuts and seeds.

### Lactose
Naturally occurring in dairy products such as milk, yogurt, soft cheeses, and ice cream.

### Fructose
Found in fruits such as apples, pears, cherries, mangoes, and honey, as well as high-fructose corn syrup.

### Polyols
Sugar alcohols like sorbitol, mannitol, xylitol, and maltitol found in certain fruits such as stone fruits (e.g., peaches, plums, cherries), as well as sugar-free gum and candies.

By identifying and avoiding high-FODMAP trigger foods, individuals can reduce the fermentable substrate available to gut bacteria, thereby alleviating symptoms and improving overall digestive health.

## Keeping a Food Diary and Tracking Symptoms

Keeping a food diary is a powerful tool for identifying trigger foods and tracking symptom patterns. The following instructions below is a guide on how to get started:

### Choose Your Format
Whether you prefer a physical notebook, a mobile app, or an online tool, select a format that suits your lifestyle and preferences.

### Record Everything You Eat and Drink
Be diligent about documenting everything you consume throughout the day, including meals, snacks, beverages, and portion sizes.

## Note Symptoms
Record any digestive symptoms you experience, such as bloating, gas, abdominal pain, diarrhea, or constipation, along with their severity and duration.

## Include Additional Factors
Consider other factors that may influence your symptoms, such as stress levels, sleep quality, exercise, medication use, and menstrual cycle for menstruating individuals.

## Review and Analyze
Periodically review your food diary to identify patterns and correlations between your dietary intake and symptoms. Look for common triggers and consider potential culprits that may be exacerbating your symptoms.

By maintaining a detailed food diary and symptom log, you can gain valuable insights into your unique trigger foods and develop a personalized approach to managing your symptoms.

# Reintroducing High-FODMAP Foods During the Challenge Phase

The challenge phase of the low-FODMAP diet involves systematically reintroducing high-FODMAP foods into your diet to assess your tolerance levels and identify individual triggers.

Below are some strategies to guide you through this process:

## Start Slowly
Begin by reintroducing one high-FODMAP food at a time in small portions, allowing several days between challenges to monitor your symptoms.

## Choose Your Foods
Select high-FODMAP foods that you miss the most or suspect may be potential triggers based on your food diary and symptom log.

## Monitor Symptoms
Pay close attention to any changes in symptoms after reintroducing a high-FODMAP food, noting the type, severity, and duration of symptoms experienced.

## Assess Tolerance
Evaluate your tolerance to each reintroduced food based on the severity and duration of symptoms. Gradually increase portion sizes or frequency of consumption if tolerated well.

## Listen to Your Body
Trust your body's signals and honor your limits. If a particular high-FODMAP food consistently triggers symptoms, consider limiting or avoiding it in the future.

The challenge phase of the low-FODMAP diet is an opportunity to gather valuable information about your individual triggers and tolerance levels. By approaching the process systematically and mindfully, you can develop a greater understanding of your digestive system and empower yourself to make informed dietary choices that support your health and well-being.

# Tracking Symptoms

Tracking symptoms is critical in the management of irritable bowel syndrome (IBS) and small intestinal bacterial overgrowth (SIBO) since it allows you to spot patterns, recognize trigger foods, and gain insights into your own digestive health.

Symptom monitoring is an effective tool for those following the low-FODMAP diet since it enables the detection of patterns and connections between food consumption and digestive symptoms.

Individuals who rigorously document symptoms might receive useful insights into their specific trigger foods, symptom triggers, and reaction to dietary changes.

This information enables people to make educated dietary decisions, customize meal plans to meet their personal needs, and improve symptom management.

Symptom monitoring also improves communication with healthcare practitioners by giving vital information that may help guide treatment options and assist collaborative decision-making.

Sharing symptom diaries with healthcare practitioners allows consumers to obtain individualized suggestions, track progress over time, and alter treatment regimens as required. Furthermore, symptom tracking promotes accountability and motivation, allowing people to take an active part in their own health and well-being.

## Symptom Tracking Methods

Effective symptom tracking requires a systematic and consistent approach. Some guidance on symptom tracking methods tailored specifically for individuals following the low-FODMAP diet are given below:

### **Journaling**

Keeping a written food diary and symptom journal is a classic method for tracking symptoms. Choose a notebook or journal to dedicate to recording your dietary intake and symptoms.

Create daily entries documenting everything you eat and drink, along with any digestive symptoms experienced, their severity, and duration.

Consider including additional factors such as stress levels, sleep quality, and exercise habits to provide context for your symptoms.

### **Mobile Apps**

In the digital age, mobile apps offer a convenient and accessible way to track symptoms on the go. There are several apps available specifically designed for tracking digestive symptoms and dietary intake.

Look for apps that allow you to input meals, log symptoms, and generate reports or summaries of your tracking data.

Some apps even offer customizable features such as reminders, meal planning tools, and integration with wearable devices for comprehensive symptom management.

### Online Tools

Online platforms and websites provide another option for symptom tracking and analysis. Explore online tools that offer customizable tracking templates, symptom charts, and data visualization features to help you identify patterns and trends in your symptoms.

Consider sharing your tracking data with healthcare providers or joining online communities for support and encouragement from others on a similar journey.

### Smart Devices

With the advent of smart devices and wearable technology, tracking symptoms has become more seamless and integrated into daily life.

Smart devices such as fitness trackers and smartwatches can monitor various health metrics, including activity levels, heart rate, and sleep patterns, which may provide valuable insights into factors influencing digestive health.

Look for devices that offer customizable tracking features and compatibility with symptom tracking apps or platforms.

## Incorporating Symptom Tracking into Your Routine

Incorporating symptom tracking into your daily routine may seem daunting at first, but with practice and consistency, it can become a valuable habit that supports your digestive health journey.

*Here are some practical tips for making symptom tracking more manageable and effective:*

### Set Reminders
Use alarms, notifications, or calendar reminders to prompt you to record your meals and symptoms at regular intervals throughout the day. Consistency is key to capturing accurate data and identifying patterns over time.

### Be Honest and Detailed
Record your dietary intake and symptoms honestly and in detail, without omitting or embellishing information. Include portion sizes, cooking methods, and ingredients to provide a comprehensive picture of your dietary habits.

### Use Keywords
Develop a set of keywords or symbols to quickly and efficiently record your symptoms. Use descriptive terms such as "bloating," "gas," "abdominal pain," "diarrhea," or "constipation" to categorize your symptoms and facilitate analysis.

### Review and Reflect
Take time to review your tracking data regularly and reflect on any patterns or trends that emerge. Look for common triggers, symptom triggers, and potential associations between dietary intake and symptoms. Consider experimenting with modifications to your diet based on your findings and evaluating the impact on your symptoms.

### Seek Support
Share your tracking data and insights with healthcare professionals, dietitians, or support groups for feedback and guidance. Collaborate with others on a similar journey to exchange tips, strategies, and encouragement for managing symptoms and optimizing digestive health.

By diligently recording dietary intake and symptoms, individuals can gain insights into their unique trigger foods, symptom triggers, and response to dietary interventions. Whether through journaling, mobile apps, online tools, or smart devices, finding a tracking method that works for you is essential for optimizing symptom management and improving overall digestive health.

## Understanding Food Labels

In this part, we look at FODMAP-related substances and additives that are widely found in processed foods, give practical techniques for reading product labels, and present a list of typical hidden sources of FODMAPs in packaged foods.

Armed with information and awareness, you may confidently navigate the shopping aisles and avoid hidden FODMAP sources that may worsen your symptoms.

Processed foods frequently contain a variety of FODMAP-containing chemicals and additives, making the low-FODMAP diet difficult to maintain.

To make educated decisions about which items to include in your diet, you should get familiar with common FODMAP-related substances and additives.

*Here are some key offenders to watch out for:*

### **Wheat-Based Ingredients**

Wheat contains high levels of fructans, making it a common trigger for individuals with IBS and SIBO. Look for ingredients such as wheat flour, wheat starch, semolina, durum wheat, and bulgur on food labels, which may indicate the presence of high-FODMAP grains.

## Onion and Garlic Powders
Onion and garlic are rich sources of fructans, often used as flavor enhancers in processed foods. Watch out for onion and garlic powders listed in ingredient lists, as they may contribute to FODMAP-related symptoms.

## High-Fructose Corn Syrup (HFCS)
HFCS is a sweetener derived from corn and is high in fructose, making it a potential trigger for individuals sensitive to fructose. Check food labels for HFCS or other corn-derived sweeteners, which may be present in a variety of processed foods and beverages.

## Sugar Alcohols
Sugar alcohols such as sorbitol, mannitol, xylitol, and maltitol are commonly used as sweeteners in sugar-free and "diet" products. These sugar alcohols can ferment in the gut, leading to gas, bloating, and diarrhea in sensitive individuals.

## Inulin and Chicory Root Extract
Inulin and chicory root extract are prebiotic fibers that are high in fructans and often added to processed foods as dietary fiber supplements. These ingredients may contribute to FODMAP-related symptoms in some individuals.

# How to Read Food Labels

Navigating food labels can be overwhelming, but with practice and attention to detail, you can become proficient at identifying potential triggers and making informed choices.

*Here are some tips for reading food labels to identify potential sources of FODMAPs:*

## Check the Ingredient List
Start by examining the ingredient list for common high-FODMAP ingredients and additives. Look for terms such as "wheat," "onion powder," "garlic powder," "high-fructose corn syrup," "sugar alcohols," "inulin," and "chicory root extract," which may indicate the presence of FODMAPs.

## Look for FODMAP-Friendly Alternatives
Seek out products that are labeled as "low-FODMAP" or "FODMAP-friendly" whenever possible. These products have undergone testing to ensure that they meet low-FODMAP criteria and are safe for individuals following the diet.

## Be Cautious of Hidden Sources
Be aware that FODMAP-related ingredients and additives may be present in unexpected places, such as condiments, sauces, salad dressings, soups, and snack foods. Take extra care to read labels carefully and avoid products that contain potential triggers.

## Watch for Serving Sizes
Pay attention to serving sizes listed on food labels, as they can impact the FODMAP content of a product. Even if a food is labeled as "low-FODMAP," consuming large portions may still trigger symptoms in some individuals.

## Use Apps and Resources

Consider using mobile apps, online databases, and resources provided by reputable organizations to help you decipher food labels and identify potential sources of FODMAPs. These tools can provide valuable information and support as you navigate the grocery aisles.

## Common Hidden Sources of FODMAPs in Packaged Foods

*To help you make informed choices while grocery shopping, here is a list of common hidden sources of FODMAPs in packaged foods:*

### Salad Dressings

Many commercial salad dressings contain onion or garlic powder as flavoring agents, making them potential triggers for individuals sensitive to FODMAPs.

### Sauces and Marinades

Barbecue sauce, teriyaki sauce, and marinades may contain high-FODMAP ingredients such as honey, garlic, or onion, which can contribute to symptoms.

### Snack Bars and Granola

Snack bars and granola often contain dried fruits, honey, or sugar alcohols as sweeteners, which may be high in FODMAPs.

### Protein Bars and Shakes

Protein bars and shakes may contain high-FODMAP ingredients such as inulin, chicory root extract, or sugar alcohols to enhance texture and flavor.

## **Cereals and Breakfast Bars**

Cereals and breakfast bars may contain wheat-based ingredients, dried fruits, or honey, which can contribute to FODMAP-related symptoms.

By being vigilant about reading food labels and avoiding hidden sources of FODMAPs, you can minimize your exposure to potential triggers and optimize symptom management on the low-FODMAP diet.

Also familiarizing yourself with common FODMAP-related ingredients and additives, using practical tips for reading food labels, and being mindful of hidden sources of FODMAPs in packaged foods, you can make informed dietary choices that support your digestive health and well-being.

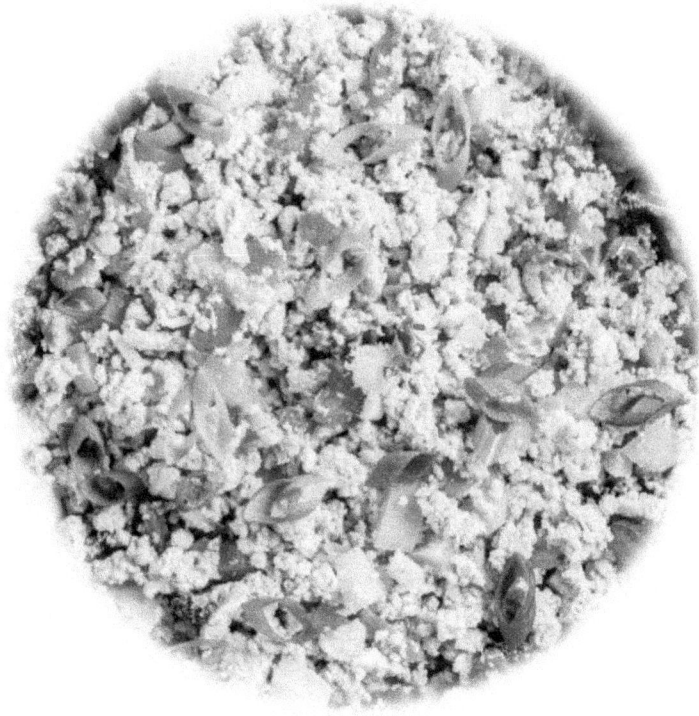

# CHAPTER TWO

## Breakfast Recipes

### Scrambled Tofu Breakfast Bowl

*Prep Time: 10 minutes | Cooking Time: 10 minutes | Servings: 2*

**Ingredients:**
- 1 block (14 oz) firm tofu, drained and crumbled
- 1 tablespoon olive oil
- 1/2 cup diced bell peppers
- 1/2 cup diced zucchini
- 1/4 teaspoon turmeric powder
- Salt and pepper to taste
- 2 cups spinach leaves
- 2 tablespoons chopped fresh chives (optional, for garnish)

**Method:**
1. Heat olive oil in a large skillet over medium heat. Add diced bell peppers and zucchini, and sauté until slightly softened, about 3-4 minutes.
2. Add crumbled tofu to the skillet, along with turmeric powder, salt, and pepper. Cook, stirring occasionally, until tofu is heated through and slightly golden, about 5-6 minutes.
3. Stir in spinach leaves and cook until wilted, about 1-2 minutes.
4. Divide the scrambled tofu mixture into serving bowls. Garnish with chopped chives if desired.
5. Serve hot and enjoy!

*Nutritional Info (per serving): Calories: 235 | Total Fat: 14g | Saturated Fat: 2g | Cholesterol: 0mg | Sodium: 305mg | Total Carbohydrates: 9g | Dietary Fiber: 3g | Sugars: 3g | Protein: 20g*

THE LOW-FODMAP DIET COOKBOOK

| **Recipe Name:**_____ |
|---|

**Date:** / /    **Time:**_____

**Rating:** ☆ ☆ ☆ ☆ ☆

| S/N | Ingredients | Adjustment |
|---|---|---|
|  |  |  |
|  |  |  |
|  |  |  |

**Cooking Experience:** _____
_____
_____
_____

**Notes:**_____
_____
_____
_____
_____
_____

# Banana Berry Smoothie Bowl

*Prep Time: 5 minutes | Cooking Time: 0 minutes | Servings: 2*

## Ingredients:

- 2 ripe bananas, peeled and frozen
- 1 cup frozen mixed berries (such as strawberries, blueberries, and raspberries)
- 1 cup lactose-free yogurt
- 1/2 cup unsweetened almond milk
- 2 tablespoons chia seeds
- 2 tablespoons shredded coconut (optional, for garnish)
- 2 tablespoons sliced almonds (optional, for garnish)
- Fresh berries for topping (optional)

## Method:

1. In a blender, combine frozen bananas, frozen mixed berries, lactose-free yogurt, almond milk, and chia seeds.
2. Blend until smooth and creamy, adding more almond milk if needed to reach your desired consistency.
3. Pour the smoothie into serving bowls.
4. Top with shredded coconut, sliced almonds, and fresh berries if desired.
5. Serve immediately and enjoy!

*Nutritional Info (per serving): Calories: 236 | Total Fat: 9g | Saturated Fat: 1g | Cholesterol: 0mg | Sodium: 66mg | Total Carbohydrates: 35g | Dietary Fiber: 8g | Sugars: 17g | Protein: 6g*

THE LOW-FODMAP DIET COOKBOOK

| Recipe Name:_____ |

*Date:* / /   *Time:*____

Rating: ☆ ☆ ☆ ☆ ☆

| S/N | Ingredients | Adjustment |
|---|---|---|
|  |  |  |
|  |  |  |
|  |  |  |
|  |  |  |

Cooking Experience: _____
_____
_____
_____

Notes:_____
_____
_____
_____
_____
_____
_____

## Quinoa Breakfast Bowl

*Prep Time: 10 minutes | Cooking Time: 15 minutes | Servings: 2*

### Ingredients:
- 1 cup quinoa, rinsed
- 2 cups water
- 1 tablespoon coconut oil
- 1/2 cup diced strawberries
- 1/2 cup blueberries
- 2 tablespoons maple syrup
- 2 tablespoons chopped walnuts
- 1 teaspoon ground cinnamon
- 1/4 teaspoon vanilla extract
- Pinch of salt

### Method:
1. In a saucepan, combine quinoa and water. Bring to a boil, then reduce heat to low, cover, and simmer for 12-15 minutes, or until quinoa is tender and water is absorbed.
2. In a separate skillet, heat coconut oil over medium heat. Add diced strawberries and blueberries, and sauté until softened, about 3-4 minutes.
3. Stir in maple syrup, chopped walnuts, ground cinnamon, vanilla extract, and a pinch of salt. Cook for an additional 1-2 minutes.
4. Divide cooked quinoa into serving bowls. Top with the berry mixture.
5. Serve warm and enjoy!

*Nutritional Info (per serving): Calories: 347 | Total Fat: 11g | Saturated Fat: 5g | Cholesterol: 0mg | Sodium: 6mg | Total Carbohydrates: 57g | Dietary Fiber: 8g | Sugars: 16g | Protein: 8g*

| Recipe Name: _____ |
|---|

*Date:*  /  /                                                    *Time:*_____

Rating: ☆ ☆ ☆ ☆ ☆

| S/N | Ingredients | Adjustment |
|---|---|---|
|  |  |  |
|  |  |  |
|  |  |  |
|  |  |  |
|  |  |  |
|  |  |  |

Cooking Experience: _____
_____
_____
_____

Notes: _____
_____
_____
_____
_____
_____

# Veggie Omelette

*Prep Time: 10 minutes | Cooking Time: 10 minutes | Servings: 2*

## Ingredients:
- 4 large eggs
- 2 tablespoons lactose-free milk
- 1 tablespoon olive oil
- 1/2 cup diced bell peppers
- 1/2 cup diced zucchini
- Salt and pepper to taste
- 2 tablespoons chopped fresh parsley (optional, for garnish)

## Method:
1. In a bowl, whisk together eggs and lactose-free milk until well combined. Season with salt and pepper to taste.
2. Heat olive oil in a non-stick skillet over medium heat. Add diced bell peppers and zucchini, and sauté until slightly softened, about 3-4 minutes.
3. Pour the egg mixture evenly over the sautéed vegetables in the skillet.
4. Cook the omelette, lifting the edges with a spatula and tilting the skillet to allow the uncooked eggs to flow underneath, until the bottom is set and the top is slightly runny, about 3-4 minutes.
5. Carefully fold the omelette in half with the spatula and cook for an additional 1-2 minutes, or until the eggs are cooked through.
6. Transfer the omelette to a serving plate. Garnish with chopped fresh parsley if desired.
7. Serve hot and enjoy!

*Nutritional Info (per serving): Calories: 229 | Total Fat: 16g | Saturated Fat: 4g | Cholesterol: 372mg | Sodium: 101mg | Total Carbohydrates: 5g | Dietary Fiber: 1g | Sugars: 3g | Protein: 15g*

| **Recipe Name:** _____ |
|---|

*Date:* / /                                    *Time:*_____

Rating: ☆ ☆ ☆ ☆ ☆

| S/N | Ingredients | Adjustment |
|---|---|---|
|   |   |   |
|   |   |   |
|   |   |   |
|   |   |   |
|   |   |   |

**Cooking Experience:** _____
_____
_____
_____

**Notes:** _____
_____
_____
_____
_____
_____
_____

# Peanut Butter Banana Overnight Oats

*Prep Time: 5 minutes | Cooking Time: 0 minutes (overnight soaking) | Servings: 2*

## Ingredients:

- 1 cup gluten-free rolled oats
- 1 cup lactose-free milk or almond milk
- 2 tablespoons smooth peanut butter
- 1 ripe banana, mashed
- 1 tablespoon maple syrup (optional)
- 1 tablespoon chia seeds
- Sliced bananas and crushed peanuts for topping (optional)

## Method:

1. In a mixing bowl, combine rolled oats, lactose-free milk, smooth peanut butter, mashed banana, maple syrup (if using), and chia seeds. Stir well to combine.
2. Divide the oat mixture evenly between two jars or containers with lids.
3. Cover the jars or containers and refrigerate overnight, or for at least 4 hours, to allow the oats to soften and absorb the liquid.
4. Before serving, give the oats a good stir. If desired, top with sliced bananas and crushed peanuts for extra flavor and texture.
5. Serve chilled and enjoy your delicious peanut butter banana overnight oats!

*Nutritional Info (per serving): Calories: 343 | Total Fat: 14g | Saturated Fat: 2g | Cholesterol: 0mg | Sodium: 70mg | Total Carbohydrates: 47g | Dietary Fiber: 8g | Sugars: 11g | Protein: 10g*

## Recipe Name:_____

*Date:* / /          *Time:*____

Rating: ☆ ☆ ☆ ☆ ☆

| S/N | Ingredients | Adjustment |
|---|---|---|
|  |  |  |
|  |  |  |
|  |  |  |
|  |  |  |
|  |  |  |

**Cooking Experience:** _____
_____
_____
_____

**Notes:**_____
_____
_____
_____
_____
_____

## Spinach and Tomato Frittata

*Prep Time: 10 minutes | Cooking Time: 20 minutes | Servings: 4*

## Ingredients:
- 6 large eggs
- 1/4 cup lactose-free milk or almond milk
- 1 tablespoon olive oil
- 1 cup baby spinach leaves
- 1 cup cherry tomatoes, halved
- Salt and pepper to taste
- 1/4 cup grated lactose-free cheese (optional)

## Method:
1. Preheat the oven to 350°F (175°C).
2. In a bowl, whisk together eggs and lactose-free milk until well combined. Season with salt and pepper to taste.
3. Heat olive oil in an oven-safe skillet over medium heat. Add baby spinach leaves and cherry tomatoes, and sauté until spinach is wilted and tomatoes are slightly softened, about 2-3 minutes.
4. Pour the egg mixture evenly over the sautéed vegetables in the skillet.
5. Cook the frittata on the stovetop for 3-4 minutes, or until the edges begin to set.
6. Sprinkle grated lactose-free cheese (if using) evenly over the top of the frittata.
7. Transfer the skillet to the preheated oven and bake for 12-15 minutes, or until the frittata is set and the top is golden brown.
8. Remove the skillet from the oven and let the frittata cool for a few minutes before slicing.
9. Slice the frittata into wedges and serve warm.

*Nutritional Info (per serving): Calories: 151 | Total Fat: 11g | Saturated Fat: 3g | Cholesterol: 285mg | Sodium: 147mg | Total Carbohydrates: 3g | Dietary Fiber: 1g | Sugars: 2g | Protein: 10g*

# Recipe Name:_____

**Date:** / /                                **Time:**_____

**Rating:** ☆ ☆ ☆ ☆ ☆

| S/N | Ingredients | Adjustment |
|-----|-------------|------------|
|     |             |            |
|     |             |            |
|     |             |            |
|     |             |            |
|     |             |            |
|     |             |            |

**Cooking Experience:** _____
_____
_____
_____

**Notes:**_____
_____
_____
_____
_____
_____
_____

## Lactose-Free Pancakes

*Prep Time: 10 minutes | Cooking Time: 15 minutes | Servings: 4*

## Ingredients:
- 1 cup gluten-free all-purpose flour
- 1 tablespoon granulated sugar
- 1 teaspoon baking powder
- 1/2 teaspoon baking soda
- 1/4 teaspoon salt
- 1 cup lactose-free milk or almond milk
- 2 large eggs
- 2 tablespoons coconut oil, melted
- 1 teaspoon vanilla extract
- Maple syrup and fresh berries for serving (optional)

## Method:
1. In a large mixing bowl, whisk together gluten-free all-purpose flour, granulated sugar, baking powder, baking soda, and salt.
2. In a separate bowl, whisk together lactose-free milk, eggs, melted coconut oil, and vanilla extract until well combined.
3. Pour the wet ingredients into the dry ingredients and stir until just combined. Be careful not to overmix.
4. Heat a non-stick skillet or griddle over medium heat. Lightly grease with coconut oil or non-stick cooking spray.
5. Pour about 1/4 cup of batter onto the skillet for each pancake. Cook until bubbles form on the surface and the edges look set, about 2-3 minutes. Flip and cook for an additional 1-2 minutes, or until golden brown and cooked through.
6. Repeat with the remaining batter, greasing the skillet as needed.
7. Serve the pancakes warm with maple syrup and fresh berries if desired.

***Nutritional Info (per serving): Calories: 244 | Total Fat: 9g | Saturated Fat: 6g | Cholesterol: 93mg | Sodium: 387mg | Total Carbohydrates: 35g | Dietary Fiber: 1g | Sugars: 5g | Protein: 6g***

## Recipe Name: _____

***Date:*** / /    ***Time:*** _____

**Rating:** ☆ ☆ ☆ ☆ ☆

| S/N | Ingredients | Adjustment |
|-----|-------------|------------|
|     |             |            |
|     |             |            |
|     |             |            |
|     |             |            |
|     |             |            |

**Cooking Experience:** _____
_____
_____
_____

**Notes:** _____
_____
_____
_____
_____
_____
_____

## Smoked Salmon and Dill Omelette

*Prep Time: 5 minutes | Cooking Time: 10 minutes | Servings: 2*

### Ingredients:
- 4 large eggs
- 2 tablespoons lactose-free milk
- 1 tablespoon olive oil
- 2 ounces smoked salmon, thinly sliced
- 2 tablespoons chopped fresh dill
- Salt and pepper to taste

### Method:
1. In a bowl, whisk together eggs and lactose-free milk until well combined. Season with salt and pepper to taste.
2. Heat olive oil in a non-stick skillet over medium heat.
3. Pour half of the egg mixture into the skillet, swirling to evenly distribute.
4. Cook the omelette for 2-3 minutes, or until the bottom is set and the top is slightly runny.
5. Arrange half of the smoked salmon slices and chopped fresh dill on one half of the omelette.
6. Carefully fold the other half of the omelette over the filling, creating a half-moon shape.
7. Cook for an additional 1-2 minutes, or until the eggs are cooked through and the smoked salmon is warmed.
8. Repeat with the remaining egg mixture and filling ingredients to make a second omelette.
9. Transfer the omelettes to serving plates and garnish with additional chopped fresh dill if desired.
10. Serve hot and enjoy!

*Nutritional Info (per serving): Calories: 230 | Total Fat: 17g | Saturated Fat: 4g | Cholesterol: 368mg | Sodium: 460mg | Total Carbohydrates: 1g | Dietary Fiber: 0g | Sugars: 1g | Protein: 18g*

| Recipe Name: |
|---|

*Date:* / /  *Time:*____

Rating: ☆ ☆ ☆ ☆ ☆

| S/N | Ingredients | Adjustment |
|---|---|---|
|  |  |  |

Cooking Experience: _____
_____
_____
_____

Notes: _____
_____
_____
_____
_____
_____
_____

## Greek Yogurt Parfait

*Prep Time: 5 minutes | Cooking Time: 0 minutes | Servings: 2*

## Ingredients:
- 1 cup lactose-free Greek yogurt
- 1/2 cup fresh strawberries, sliced
- 1/2 cup fresh blueberries
- 2 tablespoons chopped walnuts
- 2 tablespoons shredded coconut
- 1 tablespoon maple syrup (optional)
- Fresh mint leaves for garnish (optional)

## Method:
1. In two serving glasses or bowls, layer the lactose-free Greek yogurt, sliced strawberries, and blueberries.
2. Sprinkle chopped walnuts and shredded coconut over the fruit layer.
3. Drizzle with maple syrup if desired for added sweetness.
4. Garnish with fresh mint leaves for a pop of color and flavor.
5. Serve immediately and enjoy your refreshing Greek yogurt parfait!

*Nutritional Info (per serving): Calories: 227 | Total Fat: 11g | Saturated Fat: 5g | Cholesterol: 4mg | Sodium: 44mg | Total Carbohydrates: 26g | Dietary Fiber: 4g | Sugars: 19g | Protein: 8g*

# Recipe Name: _____

***Date:*** / /　　　　　　　　　　　***Time:*** _____

**Rating:** ☆ ☆ ☆ ☆ ☆

| S/N | Ingredients | Adjustment |
|---|---|---|
| | | |
| | | |
| | | |
| | | |
| | | |

**Cooking Experience:** _____
_____
_____
_____

**Notes:** _____
_____
_____
_____
_____
_____
_____

# Spinach and Tomato Breakfast Burrito

*Prep Time: 10 minutes | Cooking Time: 10 minutes | Servings: 2*

## Ingredients:
- 4 large eggs
- 2 tablespoons lactose-free milk
- Salt and pepper to taste
- 1 tablespoon olive oil
- 1 cup baby spinach leaves
- 1/2 cup cherry tomatoes, halved
- 2 gluten-free tortillas
- Salsa and sliced avocado for serving (optional)

## Method:
1. In a bowl, whisk together eggs, lactose-free milk, salt, and pepper until well combined.
2. Heat olive oil in a skillet over medium heat. Add baby spinach leaves and cherry tomatoes, and sauté until spinach is wilted and tomatoes are slightly softened, about 2-3 minutes.
3. Pour the egg mixture into the skillet with the sautéed vegetables. Cook, stirring occasionally, until the eggs are scrambled and cooked through, about 3-4 minutes.
4. Warm the gluten-free tortillas in the microwave or in a dry skillet.
5. Divide the scrambled egg mixture between the tortillas, placing it in the center of each.
6. Roll up the tortillas, folding in the sides to enclose the filling.
7. Serve the breakfast burritos with salsa and sliced avocado if desired.

*Nutritional Info (per serving): Calories: 305 | Total Fat: 18g | Saturated Fat: 4g | Cholesterol: 372mg | Sodium: 237mg | Total Carbohydrates: 20g | Dietary Fiber: 3g | Sugars: 3g | Protein: 16g*

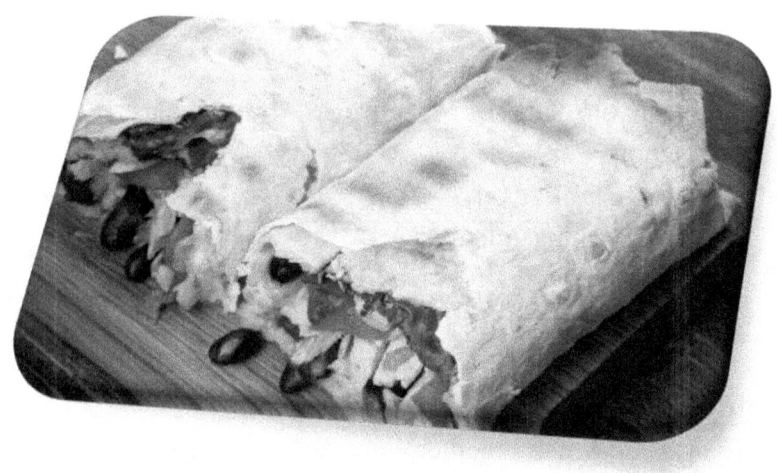

| Recipe Name:_____ |
|---|

*Date:* / /  *Time:*____

Rating: ☆ ☆ ☆ ☆ ☆

| S/N | Ingredients | Adjustment |
|---|---|---|
|  |  |  |
|  |  |  |
|  |  |  |
|  |  |  |
|  |  |  |

Cooking Experience: _____
_____
_____
_____

Notes:_____
_____
_____
_____
_____
_____
_____

# CHAPTER THREE
## Lunch Recipes

## Quinoa Salad with Lemon Herb Dressing

*Prep Time: 15 minutes | Cooking Time: 15 minutes | Servings: 4*

### Ingredients:
- 1 cup quinoa, rinsed
- 2 cups water
- 1 cup cherry tomatoes, halved
- 1 cup cucumber, diced
- 1/4 cup fresh parsley, chopped
- 2 tablespoons fresh chives, chopped
- 2 tablespoons olive oil
- 2 tablespoons lemon juice
- 1 teaspoon Dijon mustard
- Salt and pepper to taste

### Method:
1. In a medium saucepan, combine quinoa and water. Bring to a boil, then reduce heat to low, cover, and simmer for 12-15 minutes, or until quinoa is tender and water is absorbed. Remove from heat and let cool.
2. In a large mixing bowl, combine cooked quinoa, cherry tomatoes, cucumber, parsley, and chives.
3. In a small bowl, whisk together olive oil, lemon juice, Dijon mustard, salt, and pepper to make the dressing.
4. Pour the dressing over the quinoa salad and toss to coat evenly.
5. Divide the salad into serving bowls.
6. Serve chilled or at room temperature.

***Nutritional Info (per serving): Calories: 246 | Total Fat: 9g | Saturated Fat: 1g | Cholesterol: 0mg | Sodium: 11mg | Total Carbohydrates: 37g | Dietary Fiber: 5g | Sugars: 2g | Protein: 6g***

# Recipe Name:_____

*Date:* / /            *Time:*____

**Rating:** ☆ ☆ ☆ ☆ ☆

| S/N | Ingredients | Adjustment |
|-----|-------------|------------|
|     |             |            |
|     |             |            |
|     |             |            |
|     |             |            |
|     |             |            |

**Cooking Experience:** _____
_____
_____
_____

**Notes:**_____
_____
_____
_____
_____
_____
_____

## Grilled Chicken and Vegetable Skewers

*Prep Time: 20 minutes | Cooking Time: 10 minutes | Servings: 4*

### Ingredients:
- 1-pound boneless, skinless chicken breasts, cut into 1-inch cubes
- 1 zucchini, cut into 1-inch rounds
- 1 bell pepper, cut into 1-inch pieces
- 1 cup cherry tomatoes
- 1 tablespoon olive oil
- 2 tablespoons fresh lemon juice
- 2 tablespoons fresh parsley, chopped
- Salt and pepper to taste

### Method:
1. Preheat grill to medium-high heat.
2. Thread the chicken cubes, zucchini rounds, bell pepper pieces, and cherry tomatoes onto skewers, alternating between the ingredients.
3. In a small bowl, whisk together olive oil, lemon juice, chopped parsley, salt, and pepper to make the marinade.
4. Brush the marinade over the chicken and vegetable skewers, coating them evenly.
5. Place the skewers on the preheated grill and cook for 4-5 minutes per side, or until the chicken is cooked through and the vegetables are tender.
6. Remove the skewers from the grill and transfer to a serving platter.
7. Serve hot and enjoy!

*Nutritional Info (per serving): Calories: 212 | Total Fat: 7g | Saturated Fat: 1g | Cholesterol: 73mg | Sodium: 76mg | Total Carbohydrates: 7g | Dietary Fiber: 2g | Sugars: 4g | Protein: 29g*

| Recipe Name: |
|---|

*Date:*  /  /                                    *Time:*_____

Rating: ☆ ☆ ☆ ☆ ☆

| S/N | Ingredients | Adjustment |
|-----|-------------|------------|
|     |             |            |
|     |             |            |
|     |             |            |
|     |             |            |
|     |             |            |

**Cooking Experience:** _____

_____
_____
_____

**Notes:** _____

_____
_____
_____
_____
_____
_____

## Turkey and Avocado Wrap

*Prep Time: 10 minutes | Cooking Time: 0 minutes | Servings: 2*

### Ingredients:
- 4 gluten-free tortillas
- 8 slices low-sodium turkey breast
- 1 ripe avocado, sliced
- 1 cup baby spinach leaves
- 1/2 cup shredded carrots
- 1/4 cup sliced red bell pepper
- 2 tablespoons mayonnaise (check for FODMAP-friendly ingredients)
- 1 tablespoon Dijon mustard
- Salt and pepper to taste

### Method:
1. Lay out the gluten-free tortillas on a clean surface.
2. Spread mayonnaise and Dijon mustard evenly over the tortillas.
3. Divide the turkey breast slices, avocado slices, baby spinach leaves, shredded carrots, and sliced red bell pepper among the tortillas.
4. Season with salt and pepper to taste.
5. Roll up the tortillas tightly, folding in the sides to enclose the filling.
6. Slice the wraps in half diagonally, if desired, and serve immediately.

*Nutritional Info (per serving): Calories: 354 | Total Fat: 18g | Saturated Fat: 3g | Cholesterol: 50mg | Sodium: 665mg | Total Carbohydrates: 30g | Dietary Fiber: 8g | Sugars: 3g | Protein: 21g*

# Recipe Name: _____

*Date:* __ / __ / __                                    *Time:* _____

*Rating:* ☆ ☆ ☆ ☆ ☆

| S/N | Ingredients | Adjustment |
|-----|-------------|------------|
|     |             |            |
|     |             |            |
|     |             |            |
|     |             |            |
|     |             |            |

**Cooking Experience:** _____
_____
_____
_____

**Notes:** _____
_____
_____
_____
_____
_____
_____

## Quinoa and Vegetable Stir-Fry

*Prep Time: 10 minutes | Cooking Time: 15 minutes | Servings: 4*

### Ingredients:
- 1 cup quinoa, rinsed
- 2 cups water
- 1 tablespoon sesame oil
- 2 cups mixed vegetables (such as bell peppers, carrots, zucchini), chopped
- 2 tablespoons low-sodium soy sauce or tamari
- 1 tablespoon rice vinegar
- 1 tablespoon maple syrup
- 1 teaspoon grated ginger
- 2 green onions, sliced
- Sesame seeds for garnish (optional)

### Method:
1. In a medium saucepan, combine quinoa and water. Bring to a boil, then reduce heat to low, cover, and simmer for 12-15 minutes, or until quinoa is tender and water is absorbed. Remove from heat and let cool.
2. In a large skillet or wok, heat sesame oil over medium-high heat.
3. Add mixed vegetables to the skillet and stir-fry for 4-5 minutes, or until tender-crisp.
4. In a small bowl, whisk together low-sodium soy sauce or tamari, rice vinegar, maple syrup, and grated ginger to make the sauce.
5. Add cooked quinoa and sauce to the skillet with the vegetables. Stir-fry for an additional 2-3 minutes, or until everything is heated through and well combined.
6. Remove from heat and garnish with sliced green onions and sesame seeds if desired.

7. Serve hot and enjoy your flavorful quinoa and vegetable stir-fry!

*Nutritional Info (per serving): Calories: 261 | Total Fat: 6g | Saturated Fat: 1g | Cholesterol: 0mg | Sodium: 309mg | Total Carbohydrates: 45g | Dietary Fiber: 6g | Sugars: 6g | Protein: 9g*

| **Recipe Name:**_____ |

*Date:*  /  /                                    *Time:*_____

**Rating:** ☆ ☆ ☆ ☆ ☆

| S/N | Ingredients | Adjustment |
|-----|-------------|------------|
|     |             |            |
|     |             |            |
|     |             |            |
|     |             |            |
|     |             |            |
|     |             |            |

**Cooking Experience:** _____
_____
_____
_____

**Notes:**_____
_____
_____
_____
_____
_____
_____

# Tuna Salad Lettuce Wraps

*Prep Time: 10 minutes | Cooking Time: 0 minutes | Servings: 2*

## Ingredients:
- 1 can (5 oz) tuna in water, drained
- 2 tablespoons mayonnaise (check for FODMAP-friendly ingredients)
- 1 tablespoon Dijon mustard
- 1 tablespoon lemon juice
- 1/4 cup diced cucumber
- 1/4 cup diced red bell pepper
- 2 tablespoons chopped fresh parsley
- Salt and pepper to taste
- 4 large lettuce leaves (such as romaine or butter lettuce)

## Method:
1. In a mixing bowl, combine drained tuna, mayonnaise, Dijon mustard, lemon juice, diced cucumber, diced red bell pepper, and chopped fresh parsley. Stir until well combined.
2. Season with salt and pepper to taste.
3. Divide the tuna salad evenly among the lettuce leaves, spooning it onto the center of each leaf.
4. Wrap the lettuce leaves around the tuna salad, folding in the sides to enclose the filling.
5. Serve immediately and enjoy your light and refreshing tuna salad lettuce wraps!

*Nutritional Info (per serving): Calories: 196 | Total Fat: 11g | Saturated Fat: 2g | Cholesterol: 34mg | Sodium: 310mg | Total Carbohydrates: 5g | Dietary Fiber: 1g | Sugars: 2g | Protein: 20g*

# Recipe Name: _____

**Date:** / /  **Time:** _____

**Rating:** ☆ ☆ ☆ ☆ ☆

| S/N | Ingredients | Adjustment |
|---|---|---|
|  |  |  |
|  |  |  |
|  |  |  |
|  |  |  |
|  |  |  |
|  |  |  |

**Cooking Experience:** _____
_____
_____
_____

**Notes:** _____
_____
_____
_____
_____
_____
_____

## Mediterranean Quinoa Salad

*Prep Time: 15 minutes | Cooking Time: 15 minutes | Servings: 4*

### Ingredients:
- 1 cup quinoa, rinsed
- 2 cups water
- 1/4 cup Kalamata olives, pitted and sliced
- 1/4 cup diced cucumber
- 1/4 cup diced red bell pepper
- 1/4 cup crumbled feta cheese (optional)
- 2 tablespoons chopped fresh parsley
- 2 tablespoons chopped fresh mint
- 2 tablespoons extra-virgin olive oil
- 1 tablespoon red wine vinegar
- Salt and pepper to taste

### Method:
1. In a medium saucepan, combine quinoa and water. Bring to a boil, then reduce heat to low, cover, and simmer for 12-15 minutes, or until quinoa is tender and water is absorbed. Remove from heat and let cool.
2. In a large mixing bowl, combine cooked quinoa, sliced Kalamata olives, diced cucumber, diced red bell pepper, crumbled feta cheese (if using), chopped fresh parsley, and chopped fresh mint.
3. In a small bowl, whisk together extra-virgin olive oil, red wine vinegar, salt, and pepper to make the dressing.
4. Pour the dressing over the quinoa salad and toss to coat evenly.
5. Serve chilled or at room temperature.

*Nutritional Info (per serving): Calories: 246 | Total Fat: 11g | Saturated Fat: 2g | Cholesterol: 8mg | Sodium: 222mg | Total Carbohydrates: 30g | Dietary Fiber: 4g | Sugars: 1g | Protein: 7g*

| Recipe Name: _____ |

*Date:* / /                                    *Time:* ____

Rating: ☆ ☆ ☆ ☆ ☆

| S/N | Ingredients | Adjustment |
|---|---|---|
|   |   |   |
|   |   |   |
|   |   |   |
|   |   |   |
|   |   |   |

**Cooking Experience:** _____
_____
_____
_____

**Notes:** _____
_____
_____
_____
_____
_____
_____

## Grilled Chicken Salad with Lemon Vinaigrette

*Prep Time: 15 minutes | Cooking Time: 10 minutes | Servings: 2*

### Ingredients:
- 2 boneless, skinless chicken breasts
- 2 tablespoons olive oil
- Salt and pepper to taste
- 4 cups mixed salad greens (such as lettuce, spinach, arugula)
- 1 cup cherry tomatoes, halved
- 1/2 cucumber, sliced
- 1/4 cup sliced radishes
- 2 tablespoons chopped fresh basil
- 2 tablespoons chopped fresh parsley
- 2 tablespoons lemon juice
- 2 tablespoons extra-virgin olive oil

### Method:
1. Preheat grill or grill pan to medium-high heat.
2. Brush chicken breasts with olive oil and season with salt and pepper.
3. Grill chicken breasts for 4-5 minutes per side, or until cooked through and no longer pink in the center. Remove from grill and let rest for a few minutes before slicing.
4. In a large mixing bowl, combine mixed salad greens, cherry tomatoes, cucumber slices, sliced radishes, chopped fresh basil, and chopped fresh parsley.
5. In a small bowl, whisk together lemon juice and extra-virgin olive oil to make the vinaigrette.
6. Add sliced grilled chicken to the salad mixture.
7. Drizzle the lemon vinaigrette over the salad and toss to coat evenly.
8. Divide the salad into serving bowls.

9. Serve immediately and enjoy your refreshing grilled chicken salad!

*Nutritional Info (per serving): Calories: 329 | Total Fat: 21g | Saturated Fat: 3g | Cholesterol: 77mg | Sodium: 82mg | Total Carbohydrates: 10g | Dietary Fiber: 3g | Sugars: 4g | Protein: 26g*

## Recipe Name:_____

*Date:* / /           *Time:*_____

Rating: ☆ ☆ ☆ ☆ ☆

| S/N | Ingredients | Adjustment |
|---|---|---|
|   |   |   |
|   |   |   |
|   |   |   |
|   |   |   |
|   |   |   |
|   |   |   |

**Cooking Experience:** _____
_____
_____
_____

**Notes:** _____
_____
_____
_____
_____
_____
_____

# Eggplant and Tomato Quinoa Bowl

*Prep Time: 15 minutes | Cooking Time: 25 minutes | Servings: 4*

## Ingredients:
- 1 cup quinoa, rinsed
- 2 cups water
- 1 large eggplant, diced
- 2 tablespoons olive oil
- Salt and pepper to taste
- 1 cup cherry tomatoes, halved
- 1/4 cup chopped fresh basil
- 2 tablespoons balsamic vinegar
- 2 tablespoons pine nuts, toasted (optional)

## Method:
1. Preheat oven to 400°F (200°C).
2. In a medium saucepan, combine quinoa and water. Bring to a boil, then reduce heat to low, cover, and simmer for 12-15 minutes, or until quinoa is tender and water is absorbed. Remove from heat and let cool.
3. Place diced eggplant on a baking sheet. Drizzle with olive oil and season with salt and pepper. Toss to coat evenly.
4. Roast eggplant in the preheated oven for 20-25 minutes, or until tender and lightly browned, stirring halfway through.
5. In a large mixing bowl, combine cooked quinoa, roasted eggplant, cherry tomatoes, chopped fresh basil, and balsamic vinegar. Toss to combine.
6. Divide the quinoa mixture into serving bowls.
7. Sprinkle toasted pine nuts over the quinoa bowls if desired.
8. Serve warm or at room temperature.

*Nutritional Info (per serving): Calories: 254 | Total Fat: 11g | Saturated Fat: 1g | Cholesterol: 0mg | Sodium: 11mg | Total Carbohydrates: 34g | Dietary Fiber: 6g | Sugars: 3g | Protein: 7g*

# Recipe Name: _____

***Date:*** / /  ***Time:*** _____

**Rating:** ☆ ☆ ☆ ☆ ☆

| S/N | Ingredients | Adjustment |
|---|---|---|
|  |  |  |
|  |  |  |
|  |  |  |
|  |  |  |
|  |  |  |

**Cooking Experience:** _____
_____
_____
_____

**Notes:** _____
_____
_____
_____
_____
_____
_____

## Shrimp and Vegetable Stir-Fry

*Prep Time: 15 minutes | Cooking Time: 10 minutes | Servings: 2*

### Ingredients:
- 8 ounces raw shrimp, peeled and deveined
- 2 tablespoons low-sodium soy sauce or tamari
- 1 tablespoon sesame oil
- 1 tablespoon olive oil
- 1 bell pepper, thinly sliced
- 1 cup sliced zucchini
- 1 cup sliced carrots
- 1 cup broccoli florets
- 2 green onions, sliced
- 2 tablespoons chopped fresh cilantro (optional)
- Cooked rice or quinoa for serving (optional)

### Method:
1. In a bowl, marinate the shrimp in low-sodium soy sauce or tamari for 10 minutes.
2. In a large skillet or wok, heat sesame oil and olive oil over medium-high heat.
3. Add bell pepper, zucchini, carrots, and broccoli to the skillet. Stir-fry for 4-5 minutes, or until vegetables are tender-crisp.
4. Add marinated shrimp to the skillet and stir-fry for an additional 2-3 minutes, or until shrimp are pink and cooked through.
5. Stir in sliced green onions and chopped fresh cilantro, if using.
6. Serve the shrimp and vegetable stir-fry hot, either on its own or over cooked rice or quinoa.

*Nutritional Info (per serving, without rice/quinoa): Calories: 220 | Total Fat: 10g | Saturated Fat: 1g | Cholesterol: 191mg | Sodium: 883mg | Total Carbohydrates: 14g | Dietary Fiber: 4g | Sugars: 6g | Protein: 19g*

# Recipe Name: _____

*Date:* / /          *Time:* ____

Rating: ☆ ☆ ☆ ☆ ☆

| S/N | Ingredients | Adjustment |
|---|---|---|
| | | |
| | | |
| | | |
| | | |
| | | |

**Cooking Experience:** _____
_____
_____
_____

**Notes:** _____
_____
_____
_____
_____
_____
_____

# Turkey and Spinach Salad with Balsamic Vinaigrette

*Prep Time: 15 minutes | Cooking Time: 10 minutes | Servings: 2*

## Ingredients:
- 8 ounces cooked turkey breast, sliced
- 4 cups fresh spinach leaves
- 1/2 cup cherry tomatoes, halved
- 1/4 cup sliced cucumber
- 1/4 cup sliced radishes
- 2 tablespoons crumbled feta cheese (optional)
- 2 tablespoons balsamic vinegar
- 2 tablespoons extra-virgin olive oil
- Salt and pepper to taste

## Method:
1. In a large mixing bowl, combine fresh spinach leaves, cherry tomatoes, sliced cucumber, sliced radishes, and cooked turkey breast slices.
2. In a small bowl, whisk together balsamic vinegar, extra-virgin olive oil, salt, and pepper to make the vinaigrette.
3. Drizzle the balsamic vinaigrette over the salad and toss to coat evenly.
4. Divide the salad into serving bowls.
5. Sprinkle crumbled feta cheese over the salads, if using.
6. Serve immediately and enjoy your flavorful turkey and spinach salad!

*Nutritional Info (per serving): Calories: 246 | Total Fat: 13g | Saturated Fat: 2g | Cholesterol: 65mg | Sodium: 271mg | Total Carbohydrates: 9g | Dietary Fiber: 3g | Sugars: 4g | Protein: 23g*

| Recipe Name: _____ |
|---|

*Date:*  /  /                                    *Time:*____

Rating: ☆ ☆ ☆ ☆ ☆

| S/N | Ingredients | Adjustment |
|---|---|---|
|  |  |  |
|  |  |  |
|  |  |  |
|  |  |  |
|  |  |  |

Cooking Experience: _____
_____
_____
_____

Notes:_____
_____
_____
_____
_____
_____
_____

# CHAPTER FOUR

## Dinner Recipes

### Lemon Herb Baked Salmon

*Prep Time: 10 minutes | Cooking Time: 15 minutes | Servings: 4*

### Ingredients:
- 4 salmon fillets (4-6 ounces each)
- 2 tablespoons olive oil
- 2 tablespoons fresh lemon juice
- 2 cloves garlic, minced (optional, omit for low-FODMAP)
- 2 tablespoons chopped fresh parsley
- 1 tablespoon chopped fresh dill
- Salt and pepper to taste
- Lemon slices for garnish (optional)

### Method:
1. Preheat oven to 400°F (200°C). Line a baking sheet with parchment paper or aluminum foil.
2. Place salmon fillets on the prepared baking sheet.
3. In a small bowl, whisk together olive oil, lemon juice, minced garlic (if using), chopped parsley, and chopped dill.
4. Drizzle the lemon herb mixture over the salmon fillets, coating them evenly.
5. Season salmon with salt and pepper to taste.
6. Bake in the preheated oven for 12-15 minutes, or until salmon is cooked through and flakes easily with a fork.
7. Remove from oven and garnish with lemon slices if desired.
8. Serve hot with your favorite low-FODMAP side dishes.

*Nutritional Info (per serving): Calories: 279 | Total Fat: 17g | Saturated Fat: 3g | Cholesterol: 71mg | Sodium: 61mg | Total Carbohydrates: 1g | Dietary Fiber: 0g | Sugars: 0g | Protein: 30g*

THE LOW-FODMAP DIET COOKBOOK

**Recipe Name:** _____

*Date:*  /  /                               *Time:* _____

**Rating:** ☆ ☆ ☆ ☆ ☆

| S/N | Ingredients | Adjustment |
|-----|-------------|------------|
|     |             |            |
|     |             |            |
|     |             |            |
|     |             |            |
|     |             |            |
|     |             |            |

**Cooking Experience:** _____
_____
_____
_____

**Notes:** _____
_____
_____
_____
_____
_____

## Quinoa Stuffed Bell Peppers

*Prep Time: 20 minutes | Cooking Time: 30 minutes | Servings: 4*

### Ingredients:
- 4 large bell peppers (any color), halved and seeds removed
- 1 cup quinoa, rinsed
- 2 cups water or low-sodium vegetable broth
- 1 tablespoon olive oil
- 1 cup diced zucchini
- 1 cup diced eggplant
- 1 cup diced tomatoes
- 1/4 cup chopped fresh parsley
- 1/4 cup chopped fresh basil
- Salt and pepper to taste
- Grated Parmesan cheese for topping (optional)

### Method:
1. Preheat oven to 375°F (190°C). Grease a baking dish with olive oil or cooking spray.
2. In a medium saucepan, combine quinoa and water or vegetable broth. Bring to a boil, then reduce heat to low, cover, and simmer for 12-15 minutes, or until quinoa is tender and liquid is absorbed. Remove from heat and let cool slightly.
3. In a large skillet, heat olive oil over medium heat. Add diced zucchini, eggplant, and tomatoes to the skillet. Cook, stirring occasionally, for 5-6 minutes, or until vegetables are tender.
4. Stir cooked quinoa into the skillet with the cooked vegetables. Add chopped parsley and basil. Season with salt and pepper to taste. Stir to combine.
5. Arrange halved bell peppers in the prepared baking dish.
6. Spoon the quinoa and vegetable mixture evenly into each bell pepper half.

7. Cover the baking dish with aluminum foil and bake in the preheated oven for 25-30 minutes, or until bell peppers are tender.
8. If desired, sprinkle grated Parmesan cheese over the stuffed bell peppers during the last 5 minutes of baking.
9. Serve hot and enjoy your delicious quinoa stuffed bell peppers!

*Nutritional Info (per serving): Calories: 283 | Total Fat: 7g | Saturated Fat: 1g | Cholesterol: 0mg | Sodium: 28mg | Total Carbohydrates: 47g | Dietary Fiber: 8g | Sugars: 8g | Protein: 9g*

THE LOW-FODMAP DIET COOKBOOK

## Recipe Name: _____

*Date:* / /    *Time:* _____

*Rating:* ☆ ☆ ☆ ☆ ☆

| S/N | Ingredients | Adjustment |
|-----|-------------|------------|
|     |             |            |
|     |             |            |
|     |             |            |
|     |             |            |
|     |             |            |
|     |             |            |
|     |             |            |

**Cooking Experience:** _____
_____
_____
_____

**Notes:** _____
_____
_____
_____
_____
_____
_____

## Chicken and Vegetable Stir-Fry

*Prep Time: 15 minutes | Cooking Time: 15 minutes | Servings: 4*

### Ingredients:
- 1-pound boneless, skinless chicken breasts, sliced
- 2 tablespoons low-sodium soy sauce or tamari
- 1 tablespoon sesame oil
- 1 tablespoon olive oil
- 2 bell peppers (any color), sliced
- 1 cup sliced carrots
- 1 cup broccoli florets
- 1 cup sliced zucchini
- 2 tablespoons chopped green onions (green parts only)
- Cooked rice or quinoa for serving (optional)

### Method:
1. In a bowl, marinate the sliced chicken breasts in low-sodium soy sauce or tamari for 10 minutes.
2. Heat olive oil and sesame oil in a large skillet or wok over medium-high heat.
3. Add the marinated chicken to the skillet and stir-fry for 4-5 minutes, or until chicken is cooked through.
4. Add sliced bell peppers, sliced carrots, broccoli florets, and sliced zucchini to the skillet. Stir-fry for an additional 4-5 minutes, or until vegetables are tender-crisp.
5. Stir in chopped green onions and cook for 1-2 minutes more.
6. Serve the chicken and vegetable stir-fry hot, either on its own or over cooked rice or quinoa.

*Nutritional Info (per serving, without rice/quinoa): Calories: 236 | Total Fat: 8g | Saturated Fat: 1g | Cholesterol: 73mg | Sodium: 295mg | Total Carbohydrates: 9g | Dietary Fiber: 3g | Sugars: 4g | Protein: 30g*

# Recipe Name: _____

**Date:** / /     **Time:** ____

**Rating:** ☆ ☆ ☆ ☆ ☆

| S/N | Ingredients | Adjustment |
|-----|-------------|------------|
|     |             |            |
|     |             |            |
|     |             |            |
|     |             |            |
|     |             |            |

**Cooking Experience:** _____
_____
_____
_____

**Notes:** _____
_____
_____
_____
_____
_____
_____

## Baked Turkey Meatballs

*Prep Time: 15 minutes | Cooking Time: 25 minutes | Servings: 4*

### Ingredients:
- 1-pound lean ground turkey
- 1/4 cup gluten-free breadcrumbs
- 1/4 cup finely grated Parmesan cheese
- 1 egg
- 2 tablespoons chopped fresh parsley
- 1 teaspoon dried oregano
- 1/2 teaspoon garlic powder
- Salt and pepper to taste
- Low-FODMAP marinara sauce for serving

### Method:
1. Preheat oven to 400°F (200°C). Line a baking sheet with parchment paper.
2. In a large mixing bowl, combine ground turkey, gluten-free breadcrumbs, Parmesan cheese, egg, chopped parsley, dried oregano, garlic powder, salt, and pepper. Mix until well combined.
3. Roll the turkey mixture into golf ball-sized meatballs and place them on the prepared baking sheet.
4. Bake in the preheated oven for 20-25 minutes, or until meatballs are cooked through and browned on the outside.
5. Serve the baked turkey meatballs hot with low-FODMAP marinara sauce for dipping or over cooked pasta or zucchini noodles.

*Nutritional Info (per serving, without sauce or pasta): Calories: 205 | Total Fat: 9g | Saturated Fat: 3g | Cholesterol: 125mg | Sodium: 250mg | Total Carbohydrates: 4g | Dietary Fiber: 1g | Sugars: 0g | Protein: 26g*

## Recipe Name:_____

***Date:*** / /     ***Time:***_____

***Rating:*** ☆ ☆ ☆ ☆ ☆

| S/N | Ingredients | Adjustment |
|---|---|---|
|  |  |  |
|  |  |  |
|  |  |  |
|  |  |  |
|  |  |  |

**Cooking Experience:** _____
_____
_____
_____

**Notes:**_____
_____
_____
_____
_____
_____
_____

# Lemon Herb Grilled Chicken

*Prep Time: 10 minutes | Cooking Time: 15 minutes | Servings: 4*

## Ingredients:
- 4 boneless, skinless chicken breasts
- 2 tablespoons olive oil
- Zest and juice of 1 lemon
- 2 tablespoons chopped fresh parsley
- 1 tablespoon chopped fresh thyme
- Salt and pepper to taste
- Lemon wedges for serving (optional)

## Method:
1. Preheat grill to medium-high heat.
2. In a small bowl, whisk together olive oil, lemon zest, lemon juice, chopped parsley, chopped thyme, salt, and pepper.
3. Place chicken breasts in a shallow dish and pour the lemon herb marinade over them, turning to coat evenly. Let marinate for at least 10 minutes.
4. Grill chicken breasts for 6-7 minutes per side, or until cooked through and no longer pink in the center.
5. Remove from grill and let rest for a few minutes before serving.
6. Serve hot with lemon wedges on the side, if desired.

*Nutritional Info (per serving): Calories: 217 | Total Fat: 9g | Saturated Fat: 1g | Cholesterol: 96mg | Sodium: 95mg | Total Carbohydrates: 2g | Dietary Fiber: 0g | Sugars: 0g | Protein: 30g*

**Recipe Name:** _____

*Date:* / /     *Time:* _____

Rating: ☆ ☆ ☆ ☆ ☆

| S/N | Ingredients | Adjustment |
|-----|-------------|------------|
|     |             |            |
|     |             |            |
|     |             |            |
|     |             |            |
|     |             |            |

**Cooking Experience:** _____
_____
_____
_____

**Notes:** _____
_____
_____
_____
_____
_____
_____

# Spaghetti Squash with Shrimp Scampi

*Prep Time: 15 minutes | Cooking Time: 45 minutes | Servings: 4*

## Ingredients:
- 1 medium spaghetti squash
- 1 pound large shrimp, peeled and deveined
- 4 tablespoons unsalted butter
- 4 cloves garlic, minced
- Zest and juice of 1 lemon
- 2 tablespoons chopped fresh parsley
- Salt and pepper to taste
- Grated Parmesan cheese for serving (optional)

## Method:
1. Preheat oven to 375°F (190°C). Cut the spaghetti squash in half lengthwise and scoop out the seeds.
2. Place the spaghetti squash halves, cut side down, on a baking sheet lined with parchment paper. Bake for 35-40 minutes, or until tender.
3. While the spaghetti squash is baking, prepare the shrimp scampi. In a large skillet, melt butter over medium heat. Add minced garlic and cook for 1-2 minutes, or until fragrant.
4. Add shrimp to the skillet and cook for 2-3 minutes per side, or until pink and cooked through. Stir in lemon zest, lemon juice, chopped parsley, salt, and pepper.
5. Once the spaghetti squash is cooked, use a fork to scrape the flesh into strands. Divide the spaghetti squash among serving plates.
6. Top the spaghetti squash with shrimp scampi and garnish with grated Parmesan cheese, if desired.
7. Serve hot and enjoy this delicious low-FODMAP meal!

*Nutritional Info (per serving): Calories: 262 | Total Fat: 11g | Saturated Fat: 6g | Cholesterol: 194mg | Sodium: 435mg | Total Carbohydrates: 15g | Dietary Fiber: 3g | Sugars: 6g | Protein: 27g*

# Recipe Name:_____

**Date:** / /                                              **Time:**____

**Rating:** ☆ ☆ ☆ ☆ ☆

| S/N | Ingredients | Adjustment |
|-----|-------------|------------|
|     |             |            |
|     |             |            |
|     |             |            |
|     |             |            |
|     |             |            |

**Cooking Experience:** _____
_____
_____
_____

**Notes:**_____
_____
_____
_____
_____
_____
_____

# Teriyaki Glazed Salmon

*Prep Time: 10 minutes | Cooking Time: 15 minutes | Servings: 4*

## Ingredients:
- 4 salmon fillets (4-6 ounces each)
- 1/4 cup low-sodium soy sauce or tamari
- 2 tablespoons maple syrup
- 1 tablespoon rice vinegar
- 2 cloves garlic, minced (optional, omit for low-FODMAP)
- 1 teaspoon grated fresh ginger
- 1 tablespoon sesame seeds (optional, for garnish)
- Sliced green onions (green parts only) for garnish (optional)

## Method:
1. In a small bowl, whisk together low-sodium soy sauce or tamari, maple syrup, rice vinegar, minced garlic (if using), and grated fresh ginger to make the teriyaki glaze.
2. Preheat grill or grill pan to medium-high heat.
3. Brush salmon fillets with teriyaki glaze, reserving some for later use.
4. Place salmon fillets on the preheated grill and cook for 4-5 minutes per side, or until salmon is cooked through and flakes easily with a fork.
5. Brush the cooked salmon with the remaining teriyaki glaze.
6. Sprinkle sesame seeds over the glazed salmon, if using, and garnish with sliced green onions.
7. Serve hot with your favorite low-FODMAP side dishes.

*Nutritional Info (per serving): Calories: 290 | Total Fat: 15g | Saturated Fat: 3g | Cholesterol: 71mg | Sodium: 575mg | Total Carbohydrates: 8g | Dietary Fiber: 0g | Sugars: 5g | Protein: 27g*

## Recipe Name:_____

**Date:** / /                                **Time:**_____

**Rating:** ☆ ☆ ☆ ☆ ☆

| S/N | Ingredients | Adjustment |
|-----|-------------|------------|
|     |             |            |
|     |             |            |
|     |             |            |
|     |             |            |
|     |             |            |
|     |             |            |

**Cooking Experience:** _____
_____
_____
_____

**Notes:**_____
_____
_____
_____
_____
_____
_____

## Mediterranean Chicken Skewers

*Prep Time: 20 minutes | Cooking Time: 10 minutes | Servings: 4*

### Ingredients:
- 1-pound boneless, skinless chicken breasts, cut into cubes
- 2 tablespoons olive oil
- 2 tablespoons lemon juice
- 2 cloves garlic, minced (optional, omit for low-FODMAP)
- 1 teaspoon dried oregano
- 1 teaspoon paprika
- Salt and pepper to taste
- Cherry tomatoes, halved
- Red bell pepper, cut into chunks
- Zucchini, sliced
- Wooden skewers, soaked in water for 30 minutes

### Method:
1. In a bowl, combine olive oil, lemon juice, minced garlic (if using), dried oregano, paprika, salt, and pepper to make the marinade.
2. Add chicken cubes to the marinade, tossing to coat evenly. Cover and refrigerate for at least 15 minutes, or up to 1 hour.
3. Preheat grill or grill pan to medium-high heat.
4. Thread marinated chicken cubes onto wooden skewers, alternating with cherry tomatoes, red bell pepper chunks, and zucchini slices.
5. Grill chicken skewers for 4-5 minutes per side, or until chicken is cooked through and vegetables are tender.
6. Serve hot with a side salad or rice pilaf, if desired.

*Nutritional Info (per serving): Calories: 230 | Total Fat: 10g | Saturated Fat: 2g | Cholesterol: 65mg | Sodium: 160mg | Total Carbohydrates: 6g | Dietary Fiber: 2g | Sugars: 3g | Protein: 28g*

## Recipe Name: _____

*Date:*  /  /                                    *Time:* _____

Rating: ☆ ☆ ☆ ☆ ☆

| S/N | Ingredients | Adjustment |
|-----|-------------|------------|
|     |             |            |
|     |             |            |
|     |             |            |
|     |             |            |
|     |             |            |
|     |             |            |

Cooking Experience: _____
_____
_____
_____

Notes: _____
_____
_____
_____
_____
_____
_____

# Grilled Steak with Chimichurri Sauce

*Prep Time: 15 minutes | Cooking Time: 10 minutes | Servings: 4*

## Ingredients:
- 4 beef sirloin steaks (6-8 ounces each)
- Salt and pepper to taste
- 2 tablespoons olive oil
- 1/4 cup fresh parsley, chopped
- 2 tablespoons fresh oregano, chopped
- 2 tablespoons fresh cilantro, chopped
- 2 cloves garlic, minced (optional, omit for low-FODMAP)
- 1/4 cup red wine vinegar
- 1/2 cup olive oil
- 1/2 teaspoon red pepper flakes (optional)
- Lemon wedges for serving (optional)

## Method:
1. Preheat grill to medium-high heat.
2. Season steaks with salt and pepper on both sides.
3. Drizzle olive oil over the steaks and rub to coat evenly.
4. Place steaks on the grill and cook for 4-5 minutes per side for medium-rare, or to your desired level of doneness.
5. While the steaks are grilling, prepare the chimichurri sauce. In a bowl, combine chopped parsley, oregano, cilantro, minced garlic (if using), red wine vinegar, olive oil, and red pepper flakes (if using). Mix well.
6. Once the steaks are cooked, remove them from the grill and let rest for a few minutes.
7. Serve the grilled steaks with chimichurri sauce drizzled over the top.
8. Garnish with lemon wedges, if desired.

9. Serve hot and enjoy your flavorful grilled steak with chimichurri sauce!

*Nutritional Info (per serving): Calories: 428 | Total Fat: 33g | Saturated Fat: 8g | Cholesterol: 93mg | Sodium: 81mg | Total Carbohydrates: 1g | Dietary Fiber: 0g | Sugars: 0g | Protein: 31g*

| **Recipe Name:** _____ |

*Date:* / /  *Time:*_____

*Rating:* ☆ ☆ ☆ ☆ ☆

| S/N | Ingredients | Adjustment |
|-----|-------------|------------|
|     |             |            |
|     |             |            |
|     |             |            |
|     |             |            |
|     |             |            |
|     |             |            |

**Cooking Experience:** _____
_____
_____
_____

**Notes:**_____
_____
_____
_____
_____
_____
_____

## Lemon Garlic Shrimp Pasta

*Prep Time: 10 minutes | Cooking Time: 15 minutes | Servings: 4*

### Ingredients:
- 8 ounces gluten-free pasta (such as rice or quinoa pasta)
- 1 pound large shrimp, peeled and deveined
- 2 tablespoons olive oil
- 4 cloves garlic, minced (optional, omit for low-FODMAP)
- Zest and juice of 1 lemon
- Salt and pepper to taste
- 2 tablespoons chopped fresh parsley
- Grated Parmesan cheese for serving (optional)

### Method:
1. Cook gluten-free pasta according to package instructions until al dente. Drain and set aside.
2. While the pasta is cooking, heat olive oil in a large skillet over medium heat.
3. Add minced garlic to the skillet and cook for 1-2 minutes, or until fragrant.
4. Add shrimp to the skillet and cook for 2-3 minutes per side, or until pink and cooked through.
5. Stir in lemon zest, lemon juice, chopped parsley, salt, and pepper.
6. Add cooked pasta to the skillet with the shrimp and toss to combine.
7. Cook for an additional 1-2 minutes, or until heated through.
8. Serve hot with grated Parmesan cheese sprinkled over the top, if desired.
9. Enjoy your delicious lemon garlic shrimp pasta!

*Nutritional Info (per serving): Calories: 382 | Total Fat: 11g | Saturated Fat: 2g | Cholesterol: 191mg | Sodium: 243mg | Total Carbohydrates: 45g | Dietary Fiber: 2g | Sugars: 2g | Protein: 26g*

# Recipe Name: _____

*Date:* / /　　　　　　　　　　　　　*Time:*____

*Rating:* ☆ ☆ ☆ ☆ ☆

| S/N | Ingredients | Adjustment |
|-----|-------------|------------|
|     |             |            |
|     |             |            |
|     |             |            |
|     |             |            |
|     |             |            |
|     |             |            |

**Cooking Experience:** _____
_____
_____
_____

**Notes:** _____
_____
_____
_____
_____
_____
_____

# CHAPTER FIVE

## Snack Recipes

### Rice Cake with Almond Butter and Sliced Banana

*Prep Time: 5 minutes | Servings: 1*

## Ingredients:
- 1 rice cake (gluten-free)
- 1 tablespoon almond butter (or other low-FODMAP nut butter)
- 1/2 ripe banana, sliced
- *Optional:* a drizzle of maple syrup or a sprinkle of cinnamon (if tolerated)

## Method:
1. Spread almond butter evenly over the rice cake.
2. Arrange banana slices on top of the almond butter.
3. If desired, drizzle a little maple syrup over the banana slices or sprinkle with cinnamon for added flavor.
4. Enjoy your delicious and satisfying rice cake with almond butter and sliced banana!

*Nutritional Info (per serving): Calories: 170 | Total Fat: 9g | Saturated Fat: 1g | Cholesterol: 0mg | Sodium: 30mg | Total Carbohydrates: 20g | Dietary Fiber: 3g | Sugars: 8g | Protein: 4g*

| **Recipe Name:**_____ |
|---|

*Date:* / /                                    *Time:*_____

**Rating:** ☆ ☆ ☆ ☆ ☆

| S/N | Ingredients | Adjustment |
|---|---|---|
|  |  |  |
|  |  |  |
|  |  |  |
|  |  |  |
|  |  |  |

**Cooking Experience:** _____
_____
_____
_____

**Notes:**_____
_____
_____
_____
_____
_____
_____

## Mixed Berry Parfait

*Prep Time: 10 minutes | Servings: 1*

### Ingredients:
- 1/2 cup lactose-free Greek yogurt
- 1/4 cup mixed berries (such as strawberries, blueberries, and raspberries)
- 2 tablespoons gluten-free granola
- 1 tablespoon maple syrup (optional, for sweetness)
- Fresh mint leaves for garnish (optional)

### Method:
1. In a serving glass or bowl, layer lactose-free Greek yogurt, mixed berries, and gluten-free granola.
2. Repeat the layers until all ingredients are used, ending with a layer of berries on top.
3. Drizzle with maple syrup for extra sweetness, if desired.
4. Garnish with fresh mint leaves for a pop of color and flavor.
5. Serve immediately and enjoy this refreshing and nutritious mixed berry parfait!

*Nutritional Info (per serving): Calories: 180 | Total Fat: 5g | Saturated Fat: 1g | Cholesterol: 10mg | Sodium: 30mg | Total Carbohydrates: 25g | Dietary Fiber: 3g | Sugars: 15g | Protein: 11g*

| Recipe Name:_____ |
|---|

*Date:*  /  /                                    *Time:*_____

Rating: ☆ ☆ ☆ ☆ ☆

| S/N | Ingredients | Adjustment |
|---|---|---|
|  |  |  |
|  |  |  |
|  |  |  |
|  |  |  |
|  |  |  |

Cooking Experience: _____
_____
_____
_____

Notes:_____
_____
_____
_____
_____
_____
_____

## Veggie Sticks with Hummus

*Prep Time: 10 minutes | Cooking Time: 0 minutes | Servings: 2*

### Ingredients:
- 2 medium carrots, peeled and cut into sticks
- 1 medium cucumber, cut into sticks
- 2 tablespoons low-FODMAP hummus
- Fresh parsley leaves for garnish (optional)

### Method:
1. Arrange carrot and cucumber sticks on a plate or in a serving dish.
2. Serve alongside low-FODMAP hummus for dipping.
3. Garnish with fresh parsley leaves, if desired.
4. Serve immediately and enjoy this crunchy and nutritious snack!

*Nutritional Info (per serving): Calories: 80 | Total Fat: 3g | Saturated Fat: 0g | Cholesterol: 0mg | Sodium: 150mg | Total Carbohydrates: 13g | Dietary Fiber: 4g | Sugars: 4g | Protein: 2g*

| Recipe Name: _____ |
|---|

*Date:*  /  /                                    *Time:*_____

Rating: ☆ ☆ ☆ ☆ ☆

| S/N | Ingredients | Adjustment |
|---|---|---|
|  |  |  |
|  |  |  |
|  |  |  |
|  |  |  |
|  |  |  |

Cooking Experience: _____
_____
_____
_____

Notes:_____
_____
_____
_____
_____
_____
_____

# Rice Crackers with Tuna Salad

*Prep Time: 10 minutes | Cooking Time: 0 minutes | Servings: 2*

## Ingredients:
- 6 low-FODMAP rice crackers
- 1 can (5 ounces) tuna, drained
- 2 tablespoons mayonnaise (check for low-FODMAP ingredients)
- 1 teaspoon Dijon mustard
- 2 tablespoons finely chopped celery
- Salt and pepper to taste
- Fresh chives for garnish (optional)

## Method:
1. In a small bowl, combine drained tuna, mayonnaise, Dijon mustard, and chopped celery. Mix well.
2. Season tuna salad with salt and pepper to taste.
3. Spoon tuna salad onto rice crackers, dividing evenly.
4. Garnish with fresh chives, if desired, for extra flavor.
5. Serve immediately and enjoy this protein-packed and satisfying snack!

*Nutritional Info (per serving): Calories: 180 | Total Fat: 10g | Saturated Fat: 1g | Cholesterol: 30mg | Sodium: 270mg | Total Carbohydrates: 9g | Dietary Fiber: 1g | Sugars: 0g | Protein: 13g*

# Recipe Name:_____

**Date:** / /                 **Time:**_____

**Rating:** ☆ ☆ ☆ ☆ ☆

| S/N | Ingredients | Adjustment |
|---|---|---|
|  |  |  |
|  |  |  |
|  |  |  |

**Cooking Experience:** _____

_____
_____
_____

**Notes:**_____

_____
_____
_____
_____
_____
_____

# Berry Smoothie Bowl

*Prep Time: 5 minutes | Cooking Time: 0 minutes | Servings: 1*

## Ingredients:

- 1 cup lactose-free Greek yogurt
- 1/2 cup frozen mixed berries (such as strawberries, blueberries, and raspberries)
- 1 tablespoon chia seeds
- 1 tablespoon unsweetened shredded coconut
- Fresh berries for topping (optional)
- Granola for topping (optional)

## Method:

1. In a blender, combine lactose-free Greek yogurt and frozen mixed berries. Blend until smooth.
2. Pour the berry yogurt mixture into a bowl.
3. Sprinkle chia seeds and unsweetened shredded coconut over the top.
4. Add fresh berries and granola as desired for extra flavor and texture.
5. Serve immediately and enjoy this refreshing and nutritious smoothie bowl!

*Nutritional Info (per serving): Calories: 280 | Total Fat: 12g | Saturated Fat: 5g | Cholesterol: 10mg | Sodium: 85mg | Total Carbohydrates: 23g | Dietary Fiber: 8g | Sugars: 13g | Protein: 20g*

# Recipe Name:_____

*Date:* / /  *Time:*____

Rating: ☆ ☆ ☆ ☆ ☆

| S/N | Ingredients | Adjustment |
|-----|-------------|------------|
|     |             |            |
|     |             |            |
|     |             |            |
|     |             |            |
|     |             |            |

Cooking Experience: _____

_____
_____
_____

Notes:_____

_____
_____
_____
_____
_____
_____

## Turkey and Cheese Roll-Ups

*Prep Time: 10 minutes | Cooking Time: 0 minutes | Servings: 2*

### Ingredients:
- 4 slices low-FODMAP deli turkey
- 2 slices lactose-free Swiss cheese (or other low-FODMAP cheese)
- 1/2 cup baby spinach leaves
- 1 tablespoon Dijon mustard
- Toothpicks for securing roll-ups

### Method:
1. Lay out the slices of low-FODMAP deli turkey on a clean surface.
2. Place a slice of lactose-free Swiss cheese on each turkey slice.
3. Top each slice of cheese with baby spinach leaves.
4. Spread Dijon mustard evenly over the baby spinach leaves.
5. Roll up each turkey slice tightly and secure with toothpicks.
6. Slice each roll-up into bite-sized pieces.
7. Serve immediately and enjoy these protein-packed and flavorful roll-ups!

*Nutritional Info (per serving): Calories: 150 | Total Fat: 8g | Saturated Fat: 4g | Cholesterol: 50mg | Sodium: 500mg | Total Carbohydrates: 2g | Dietary Fiber: 1g | Sugars: 0g | Protein: 18g*

**Recipe Name:**_____

*Date:*  /  /                              *Time:*_____

Rating: ☆ ☆ ☆ ☆ ☆

| S/N | Ingredients | Adjustment |
|-----|-------------|------------|
|     |             |            |
|     |             |            |
|     |             |            |
|     |             |            |
|     |             |            |
|     |             |            |

**Cooking Experience:** _____
_____
_____
_____

**Notes:**_____
_____
_____
_____
_____
_____
_____

# Cucumber and Tomato Salad

*Prep Time: 10 minutes | Cooking Time: 0 minutes | Servings: 2*

## Ingredients:
- 1 large cucumber, diced
- 1 cup cherry tomatoes, halved
- 2 tablespoons chopped fresh basil
- 1 tablespoon extra-virgin olive oil
- 1 tablespoon balsamic vinegar
- Salt and pepper to taste

## Method:
1. In a mixing bowl, combine diced cucumber, halved cherry tomatoes, and chopped fresh basil.
2. Drizzle extra virgin olive oil and balsamic vinegar over the salad.
3. Season with salt and pepper to taste.
4. Toss everything together until well combined.
5. Serve immediately or refrigerate until ready to eat.
6. Enjoy this refreshing and light cucumber and tomato salad as a healthy snack option!

*Nutritional Info (per serving): Calories: 80 | Total Fat: 6g | Saturated Fat: 1g | Cholesterol: 0mg | Sodium: 10mg | Total Carbohydrates: 6g | Dietary Fiber: 2g | Sugars: 3g | Protein: 1g*

# Recipe Name: _____

***Date:*** / /                                              ***Time:*** _____

**Rating:** ☆ ☆ ☆ ☆ ☆

| S/N | Ingredients | Adjustment |
|-----|-------------|------------|
|     |             |            |
|     |             |            |
|     |             |            |
|     |             |            |
|     |             |            |

**Cooking Experience:** _____
_____
_____
_____

**Notes:** _____
_____
_____
_____
_____
_____
_____

# Rice Cake with Avocado and Radish

*Prep Time: 5 minutes | Cooking Time: 0 minutes | Servings: 1*

## Ingredients:
- 1 rice cake (plain or lightly salted)
- 1/4 ripe avocado, mashed
- 2 radishes, thinly sliced
- 1 teaspoon lemon juice
- Salt and pepper to taste
- Red pepper flakes for garnish (optional)

## Method:
1. Spread mashed avocado evenly over the rice cake.
2. Arrange thinly sliced radishes on top of the avocado.
3. Drizzle lemon juice over the radishes.
4. Season with salt, pepper, and red pepper flakes (if using) to taste.
5. Serve immediately and enjoy this simple yet flavorful rice cake snack!

*Nutritional Info (per serving): Calories: 110 | Total Fat: 7g | Saturated Fat: 1g | Cholesterol: 0mg | Sodium: 70mg | Total Carbohydrates: 11g | Dietary Fiber: 4g | Sugars: 0g | Protein: 2g*

| Recipe Name: _____ |
|---|

*Date:* __ / __ / __                              *Time:* _____

Rating: ☆ ☆ ☆ ☆ ☆

| S/N | Ingredients | Adjustment |
|---|---|---|
|  |  |  |
|  |  |  |
|  |  |  |
|  |  |  |
|  |  |  |

Cooking Experience: _____
_____
_____
_____

Notes: _____
_____
_____
_____
_____
_____

# Turkey and Cucumber Roll-Ups

*Prep Time: 10 minutes | Cooking Time: 0 minutes | Servings: 2*

## Ingredients:
- 4 slices low-FODMAP deli turkey
- 1/2 cucumber, cut into thin strips
- 2 tablespoons cream cheese (check for low-FODMAP ingredients)
- Fresh chives, chopped, for garnish (optional)

## Method:
1. Lay out the slices of low-FODMAP deli turkey on a clean surface.
2. Spread cream cheese evenly over each turkey slice.
3. Place cucumber strips on top of the cream cheese along one edge of each turkey slice.
4. Roll up the turkey slices tightly, starting from the edge with the cucumber strips.
5. Secure each roll-up with toothpicks.
6. Sprinkle chopped fresh chives over the top for garnish, if desired.
7. Serve immediately and enjoy these tasty and protein-packed roll-ups!

*Nutritional Info (per serving): Calories: 110 | Total Fat: 6g | Saturated Fat: 3g | Cholesterol: 25mg | Sodium: 220mg | Total Carbohydrates: 2g | Dietary Fiber: 0g | Sugars: 1g | Protein: 12g*

| Recipe Name:_____ |

*Date:* / /     *Time:*____

Rating: ☆ ☆ ☆ ☆ ☆

| S/N | Ingredients | Adjustment |
|-----|-------------|------------|
|     |             |            |
|     |             |            |
|     |             |            |
|     |             |            |
|     |             |            |
|     |             |            |
|     |             |            |

**Cooking Experience:** _____
_____
_____
_____

**Notes:** _____
_____
_____
_____
_____
_____
_____

# Mixed Nuts and Seeds Snack Mix

*Prep Time: 5 minutes | Cooking Time: 0 minutes | Servings: 2*

## Ingredients:
- 1/4 cup almonds
- 1/4 cup walnuts
- 1/4 cup pumpkin seeds
- 1/4 cup sunflower seeds
- 1 tablespoon olive oil
- 1 teaspoon dried oregano
- 1/2 teaspoon paprika
- Salt to taste

## Method:
1. In a dry skillet, toast almonds, walnuts, pumpkin seeds, and sunflower seeds over medium heat for 3-4 minutes, stirring occasionally, until lightly golden and fragrant.
2. Remove from heat and let cool.
3. Transfer the toasted nuts and seeds to a mixing bowl.
4. Drizzle olive oil over the nuts and seeds, tossing to coat evenly.
5. Sprinkle dried oregano, paprika, and salt over the mixture, stirring until well combined.
6. Divide the snack mix into individual serving portions.
7. Serve immediately or store in an airtight container for later enjoyment.
8. Enjoy this crunchy and flavorful mixed nuts and seeds snack mix!

*Nutritional Info (per serving): Calories: 280 | Total Fat: 25g | Saturated Fat: 3g | Cholesterol: 0mg | Sodium: 10mg | Total Carbohydrates: 9g | Dietary Fiber: 5g | Sugars: 1g | Protein: 10g*

| **Recipe Name:** _____ |

*Date:*  /  /                              *Time:* _____

Rating: ☆ ☆ ☆ ☆ ☆

| S/N | Ingredients | Adjustment |
|-----|-------------|------------|
|     |             |            |
|     |             |            |
|     |             |            |
|     |             |            |
|     |             |            |

**Cooking Experience:** _____
_____
_____
_____

**Notes:** _____
_____
_____
_____
_____
_____
_____

# CHAPTER SIX

## Dessert Recipes

### Chocolate Banana Nice Cream

*Prep Time: 5 minutes | Cooking Time: 0 minutes | Servings: 2*

**Ingredients:**
- 2 ripe bananas, sliced and frozen
- 2 tablespoons unsweetened cocoa powder
- 1/4 teaspoon vanilla extract
- 2 tablespoons lactose-free milk (or other low-FODMAP milk)
- 1 tablespoon dark chocolate chips (optional, for garnish)
- Fresh berries for topping (optional)

**Method:**
1. Place the frozen banana slices in a blender or food processor.
2. Add unsweetened cocoa powder, vanilla extract, and lactose-free milk to the blender.
3. Blend until smooth and creamy, scraping down the sides as needed.
4. Transfer the chocolate banana nice cream to serving bowls.
5. If desired, garnish with dark chocolate chips and fresh berries.
6. Serve immediately and enjoy this delicious and guilt-free chocolate treat!

*Nutritional Info (per serving): Calories: 120 | Total Fat: 1g | Saturated Fat: 0g | Cholesterol: 0mg | Sodium: 5mg | Total Carbohydrates: 30g | Dietary Fiber: 4g | Sugars: 15g | Protein: 2g*

# Recipe Name: _____

*Date:* / /                                        *Time:* _____

Rating: ☆ ☆ ☆ ☆ ☆

| S/N | Ingredients | Adjustment |
|-----|-------------|------------|
|     |             |            |
|     |             |            |
|     |             |            |
|     |             |            |
|     |             |            |

Cooking Experience: _____
_____
_____
_____

Notes: _____
_____
_____
_____
_____
_____
_____

# Coconut Berry Chia Pudding

*Prep Time: 5 minutes (+ 2 hours chilling time) | Cooking Time: 0 minutes | Servings: 2*

## Ingredients:

- 1 cup lactose-free coconut milk (or other low-FODMAP milk)
- 1/4 cup chia seeds
- 1 tablespoon maple syrup (optional, for sweetness)
- 1/2 cup mixed berries (such as strawberries, blueberries, and raspberries)
- Unsweetened shredded coconut for garnish (optional)

## Method:

1. In a mixing bowl, combine lactose-free coconut milk, chia seeds, and maple syrup (if using). Stir well to combine.
2. Cover the bowl and refrigerate for at least 2 hours, or until the chia pudding has thickened.
3. Once the chia pudding has set, divide it between serving glasses or bowls.
4. Top each serving with mixed berries and unsweetened shredded coconut, if desired.
5. Serve chilled and enjoy this creamy and nutritious coconut berry chia pudding!

*Nutritional Info (per serving): Calories: 180 | Total Fat: 11g | Saturated Fat: 2g | Cholesterol: 0mg | Sodium: 10mg | Total Carbohydrates: 20g | Dietary Fiber: 8g | Sugars: 8g | Protein: 4g*

| Recipe Name: _____ |
|---|

*Date:* / /  *Time:*____

Rating: ☆☆☆☆☆

| S/N | Ingredients | Adjustment |
|---|---|---|
|  |  |  |
|  |  |  |
|  |  |  |
|  |  |  |
|  |  |  |
|  |  |  |

Cooking Experience: _____
_____
_____
_____

Notes: _____
_____
_____
_____
_____
_____
_____

# Peanut Butter Banana Bites

*Prep Time: 10 minutes | Cooking Time: 0 minutes | Servings: 2*

## Ingredients:
- 1 large ripe banana
- 2 tablespoons peanut butter (or other low-FODMAP nut butter)
- 2 tablespoons unsweetened shredded coconut
- 2 tablespoons dark chocolate chips (optional, for garnish)

## Method:
1. Peel the banana and slice it into thick rounds.
2. Spread peanut butter on half of the banana slices.
3. Place the remaining banana slices on top to create little banana sandwiches.
4. Roll the edges of each banana bite in unsweetened shredded coconut.
5. If desired, melt the dark chocolate chips and drizzle over the top of the banana bites for extra indulgence.
6. Serve immediately or refrigerate until ready to enjoy.
7. Enjoy these peanut butter banana bites as a tasty and satisfying dessert!

*Nutritional Info (per serving): Calories: 180 | Total Fat: 12g | Saturated Fat: 4g | Cholesterol: 0mg | Sodium: 30mg | Total Carbohydrates: 18g | Dietary Fiber: 3g | Sugars: 10g | Protein: 4g*

# Recipe Name: _____

***Date:*** / /            ***Time:*** _____

**Rating:** ☆ ☆ ☆ ☆ ☆

| S/N | Ingredients | Adjustment |
|-----|-------------|------------|
|     |             |            |
|     |             |            |
|     |             |            |
|     |             |            |
|     |             |            |

**Cooking Experience:** _____

_____
_____
_____

**Notes:** _____

_____
_____
_____
_____
_____
_____

# Lemon Blueberry Yogurt Popsicles

*Prep Time: 5 minutes (+ freezing time) | Cooking Time: 0 minutes | Servings: 4*

## Ingredients:

- 1 cup lactose-free Greek yogurt
- 1/4 cup fresh blueberries
- Zest and juice of 1 lemon
- 2 tablespoons maple syrup (optional, for sweetness)

## Method:

1. In a mixing bowl, combine lactose-free Greek yogurt, fresh blueberries, lemon zest, lemon juice, and maple syrup (if using). Stir well to combine.
2. Spoon the yogurt mixture into popsicle molds, filling each mold to the top.
3. Insert popsicle sticks into the center of each mold.
4. Freeze the popsicles for at least 4 hours, or until completely frozen.
5. Once frozen, remove the popsicles from the molds and serve immediately.
6. Enjoy these refreshing and tangy lemon blueberry yogurt popsicles as a delightful summer treat!

*Nutritional Info (per serving): Calories: 70 | Total Fat: 2g | Saturated Fat: 1g | Cholesterol: 5mg | Sodium: 20mg | Total Carbohydrates: 8g | Dietary Fiber: 1g | Sugars: 6g | Protein: 6g*

# Recipe Name: _____

*Date:* _ / _ / _   *Time:* _____

Rating: ☆ ☆ ☆ ☆ ☆

| S/N | Ingredients | Adjustment |
|-----|-------------|------------|
|     |             |            |
|     |             |            |
|     |             |            |
|     |             |            |
|     |             |            |

Cooking Experience: _____
_____
_____
_____

Notes: _____
_____
_____
_____
_____
_____
_____

# Raspberry Coconut Chia Pudding Cups

*Prep Time: 10 minutes (+ chilling time) | Cooking Time: 0 minutes | Servings: 2*

## Ingredients:
- 1 cup lactose-free coconut milk (or other low-FODMAP milk)
- 1/4 cup chia seeds
- 1 tablespoon maple syrup (optional, for sweetness)
- 1/4 cup fresh raspberries
- 2 tablespoons unsweetened shredded coconut

## Method:
1. In a mixing bowl, combine lactose-free coconut milk, chia seeds, and maple syrup (if using). Stir well to combine.
2. Cover the bowl and refrigerate for at least 2 hours, or until the chia pudding has thickened.
3. Once the chia pudding has set, divide it between serving cups.
4. Top each cup with fresh raspberries and unsweetened shredded coconut.
5. Serve chilled and enjoy these creamy and flavorful raspberry coconut chia pudding cups!

*Nutritional Info (per serving): Calories: 180 | Total Fat: 11g | Saturated Fat: 5g | Cholesterol: 0mg | Sodium: 10mg | Total Carbohydrates: 19g | Dietary Fiber: 10g | Sugars: 6g | Protein: 4g*

# Recipe Name: _____

**Date:** / /            **Time:** _____

**Rating:** ☆ ☆ ☆ ☆ ☆

| S/N | Ingredients | Adjustment |
|---|---|---|
|  |  |  |
|  |  |  |
|  |  |  |
|  |  |  |
|  |  |  |

**Cooking Experience:** _____
_____
_____
_____

**Notes:** _____
_____
_____
_____
_____
_____
_____

## Chocolate Peanut Butter Energy Balls

*Prep Time: 15 minutes (+ chilling time) | Cooking Time: 0 minutes | Servings: 12*

### Ingredients:
- 1 cup rolled oats
- 1/4 cup unsweetened cocoa powder
- 1/4 cup peanut butter (or other low-FODMAP nut butter)
- 1/4 cup maple syrup
- 1 teaspoon vanilla extract
- Pinch of salt
- 2 tablespoons unsweetened shredded coconut (for coating)

### Method:
1. In a mixing bowl, combine rolled oats, unsweetened cocoa powder, peanut butter, maple syrup, vanilla extract, and a pinch of salt. Mix well until the mixture is sticky and holds together.
2. Roll the mixture into tablespoon-sized balls using your hands.
3. Roll each ball in unsweetened shredded coconut to coat.
4. Place the energy balls on a baking sheet lined with parchment paper.
5. Refrigerate the energy balls for at least 30 minutes, or until firm.
6. Once chilled, transfer the energy balls to an airtight container and store in the refrigerator until ready to eat.
7. Enjoy these chocolate peanut butter energy balls as a satisfying and nutritious snack or dessert!

*Nutritional Info (per serving - 1 energy ball): Calories: 90 | Total Fat: 4g | Saturated Fat: 1g | Cholesterol: 0mg | Sodium: 20mg | Total Carbohydrates: 12g | Dietary Fiber: 2g | Sugars: 5g | Protein: 3g*

| **Recipe Name:**_____ |
|---|

*Date:* / /                                    *Time:*_____

Rating: ☆ ☆ ☆ ☆ ☆

| S/N | Ingredients | Adjustment |
|---|---|---|
|  |  |  |
|  |  |  |
|  |  |  |
|  |  |  |
|  |  |  |

**Cooking Experience:** _____
_____
_____
_____

**Notes:**_____
_____
_____
_____
_____
_____
_____

## Almond Butter Chocolate Chip Cookies

*Prep Time: 15 minutes | Cooking Time: 10 minutes | Servings: 12 cookies*

### Ingredients:
- 1 cup almond flour
- 1/4 cup almond butter (or other low-FODMAP nut butter)
- 1/4 cup maple syrup
- 1/2 teaspoon vanilla extract
- 1/4 teaspoon baking soda
- Pinch of salt
- 1/4 cup dark chocolate chips

### Method:
1. Preheat the oven to 350°F (175°C) and line a baking sheet with parchment paper.
2. In a mixing bowl, combine almond flour, almond butter, maple syrup, vanilla extract, baking soda, and a pinch of salt. Mix until well combined.
3. Fold in the dark chocolate chips until evenly distributed throughout the dough.
4. Using a tablespoon, scoop out portions of dough and roll them into balls. Place them on the prepared baking sheet and flatten them slightly with your palm.
5. Bake in the preheated oven for 10-12 minutes, or until the edges are golden brown.
6. Allow the cookies to cool on the baking sheet for a few minutes before transferring them to a wire rack to cool completely.
7. Enjoy these almond butter chocolate chip cookies as a delicious and satisfying dessert!

*Nutritional Info (per serving - 1 cookie): Calories: 120 | Total Fat: 8g | Saturated Fat: 1g | Cholesterol: 0mg | Sodium: 50mg | Total Carbohydrates: 10g | Dietary Fiber: 1g | Sugars: 6g | Protein: 3g*

| Recipe Name:_____ |
|---|

*Date:*  /  /                                         *Time:*_____

Rating: ☆ ☆ ☆ ☆ ☆

| S/N | Ingredients | Adjustment |
|---|---|---|
|  |  |  |
|  |  |  |
|  |  |  |
|  |  |  |
|  |  |  |
|  |  |  |
|  |  |  |

**Cooking Experience:** _____
_____
_____

**Notes:**_____
_____
_____
_____
_____
_____

## Mixed Berry Frozen Yogurt Bark

*Prep Time: 10 minutes (+ freezing time) | Cooking Time: 0 minutes | Servings: 6 servings*

### Ingredients:
- 2 cups lactose-free Greek yogurt
- 1 tablespoon maple syrup
- 1/2 cup mixed berries (such as strawberries, blueberries, and raspberries)
- 2 tablespoons unsweetened shredded coconut

### Method:
1. Line a baking sheet with parchment paper and set aside.
2. In a mixing bowl, combine lactose-free Greek yogurt and maple syrup. Mix until well combined.
3. Spread the yogurt mixture evenly onto the prepared baking sheet, about 1/4 inch thick.
4. Sprinkle mixed berries and unsweetened shredded coconut over the yogurt layer, pressing them gently into the surface.
5. Place the baking sheet in the freezer and freeze for at least 2 hours, or until the yogurt bark is firm.
6. Once frozen, break the yogurt bark into pieces using your hands or a knife.
7. Serve immediately and enjoy this refreshing and nutritious mixed berry frozen yogurt bark!

*Nutritional Info (per serving): Calories: 80 | Total Fat: 3g | Saturated Fat: 2g | Cholesterol: 5mg | Sodium: 20mg | Total Carbohydrates: 9g | Dietary Fiber: 1g | Sugars: 6g | Protein: 5g*

# Recipe Name: _____

**Date:** / /  **Time:** _____

**Rating:** ☆ ☆ ☆ ☆ ☆

| S/N | Ingredients | Adjustment |
|-----|-------------|------------|
|     |             |            |
|     |             |            |
|     |             |            |
|     |             |            |
|     |             |            |

**Cooking Experience:** _____
_____
_____
_____

**Notes:** _____
_____
_____
_____
_____
_____
_____

## Lemon Coconut Energy Bites

*Prep Time: 15 minutes | Cooking Time: 0 minutes | Servings: 12 bites*

### Ingredients:
- 1 cup unsweetened shredded coconut, plus extra for coating
- 1/2 cup almond flour
- Zest of 1 lemon
- 2 tablespoons lemon juice
- 1/4 cup maple syrup
- 1 tablespoon coconut oil, melted
- 1/2 teaspoon vanilla extract
- Pinch of salt

### Method:
1. In a food processor, combine unsweetened shredded coconut, almond flour, lemon zest, lemon juice, maple syrup, melted coconut oil, vanilla extract, and a pinch of salt. Pulse until the mixture comes together and forms a sticky dough.
2. Roll the dough into tablespoon-sized balls.
3. Roll each ball in extra shredded coconut to coat.
4. Place the coated balls on a baking sheet lined with parchment paper.
5. Refrigerate the energy bites for at least 30 minutes to firm up.
6. Once chilled, serve and enjoy these zesty and refreshing lemon coconut energy bites!

*Nutritional Info (per serving - 1 bite): Calories: 90 | Total Fat: 7g | Saturated Fat: 5g | Cholesterol: 0mg | Sodium: 10mg | Total Carbohydrates: 6g | Dietary Fiber: 2g | Sugars: 4g | Protein: 1g*

| Recipe Name: _____ |
|---|

**Date:** / /     **Time:** ____

**Rating:** ☆ ☆ ☆ ☆ ☆

| S/N | Ingredients | Adjustment |
|---|---|---|
|  |  |  |
|  |  |  |
|  |  |  |
|  |  |  |
|  |  |  |

**Cooking Experience:** _____
_____
_____
_____

**Notes:** _____
_____
_____
_____
_____
_____
_____

## Chocolate Almond Butter Rice Crispy Treats

*Prep Time: 10 minutes | Cooking Time: 5 minutes | Servings: 9 squares*

### Ingredients:

- 3 cups gluten-free rice cereal
- 1/2 cup almond butter (or other low-FODMAP nut butter)
- 1/4 cup maple syrup
- 1/4 cup unsweetened cocoa powder
- 1/4 cup coconut oil
- 1/2 teaspoon vanilla extract
- Pinch of salt

### Method:

1. In a large mixing bowl, add gluten-free rice cereal.
2. In a small saucepan over low heat, combine almond butter, maple syrup, unsweetened cocoa powder, coconut oil, vanilla extract, and a pinch of salt. Stir until the mixture is smooth and well combined.
3. Pour the chocolate mixture over the rice cereal and gently fold until the cereal is evenly coated.
4. Transfer the mixture to a parchment-lined 8x8-inch baking dish and press down firmly to create an even layer.
5. Refrigerate the mixture for at least 1 hour, or until firm.
6. Once chilled, cut into squares and serve these decadent chocolate almond butter rice crispy treats!

*Nutritional Info (per serving - 1 square): Calories: 230 | Total Fat: 14g | Saturated Fat: 7g | Cholesterol: 0mg | Sodium: 40mg | Total Carbohydrates: 23g | Dietary Fiber: 2g | Sugars: 10g | Protein: 4g*

# Recipe Name: _____

*Date:*  /  /                                    *Time:* _____

*Rating:* ☆ ☆ ☆ ☆ ☆

| S/N | Ingredients | Adjustment |
|-----|-------------|------------|
|     |             |            |
|     |             |            |
|     |             |            |
|     |             |            |
|     |             |            |
|     |             |            |

**Cooking Experience:** _____
_____
_____
_____

**Notes:** _____
_____
_____
_____
_____
_____
_____

# CHAPTER SEVEN
## Shopping List

### Produce
- Bananas
- Blueberries
- Raspberries
- Strawberries
- Lemons
- Cucumber
- Cherry tomatoes
- Fresh basil
- Fresh chives
- Avocado
- Mixed berries (for example, strawberries, blueberries, raspberries)
- Radishes

### Dairy and Alternatives
- Lactose-free Greek yogurt
- Lactose-free coconut milk
- Lactose-free milk
- Cream cheese (check for low-FODMAP ingredients)
- Butter or lactose-free butter

### Meat and Protein
- Low-FODMAP deli turkey slices
- Eggs

## Pantry Staples
- Rolled oats
- Almond flour
- Almonds
- Walnuts
- Pumpkin seeds
- Sunflower seeds
- Chia seeds
- Rice cakes
- Rice cereal (gluten-free)
- Dark chocolate chips
- Unsweetened cocoa powder
- Maple syrup
- Olive oil
- Balsamic vinegar
- Vanilla extract
- Salt
- Pepper
- Red pepper flakes
- Dried oregano
- Paprika
- Shredded unsweetened coconut

## Condiments and Sauces
- Peanut butter or other low-FODMAP nut butter
- Almond butter or other low-FODMAP nut butter

## **Bakery and Bread**
- Rice cakes

## **Frozen**
- Frozen banana slices

## **Others**
- Toothpicks

*Thank you for joining us on this Low-FODMAP journey!*
*Your commitment to your health is truly inspiring. We hope these recipes and insights bring you comfort and joy on your path to digestive wellness.*
*Wishing you delicious meals, vibrant health, and a life filled with abundance. Thank you for reading!*

www.ingramcontent.com/pod-product-compliance
Lightning Source LLC
Chambersburg PA
CBHW071053240526
45471CB00015B/1854